SPARTAN UP!

SPARTAN UP!

A TAKE-NO-PRISONERS GUIDE
TO OVERCOMING OBSTACLES
AND ACHIEVING PEAK
PERFORMANCE IN LIFE

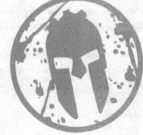

Joe De Sena

with **JEFF O'CONNELL**

MARINER BOOKS
HOUGHTON MIFFLIN HARCOURT
BOSTON   NEW YORK

First Mariner Books edition 2016

Copyright © 2014 by Spartan Race, Inc.

For information about permission to reproduce selections from
this book, write to trade.permissions@hmco.com or to Permissions,
Houghton Mifflin Harcourt Publishing Company, 3 Park Avenue,
19th Floor, New York, New York 10016.

www.hmhco.com

Library of Congress Cataloging-in-Publication Data
De Sena, Joe, date.
Spartan up! : a take-no-prisoners guide to overcoming obstacles and achieving peak
performance in life / Joe De Sena with Jeff O'Connell.
pages cm
ISBN 978-0-544-28617-7 (hardcover) ISBN 978-0-544-57021-4 (pbk.)
1. Obstacle racing. 2. Success—Psychological aspects. I. O'Connell, Jeff, date. II. Title.
GV1067.D4 2014
796.42'6 — dc23
2013050982

Book design by Brian Moore

Printed in the United States of America

23 24 25 26 27 LBC 11 10 9 8 7

THIS BOOK PRESENTS THE IDEAS OF ITS AUTHOR. YOU SHOULD CONSULT
WITH A PROFESSIONAL HEALTH CARE PROVIDER BEFORE COMMENCING
ANY DIET OR EXERCISE PLAN. THE AUTHOR AND THE PUBLISHER DISCLAIM
LIABILITY FOR ANY ADVERSE EFFECTS RESULTING DIRECTLY OR INDIRECTLY
FROM INFORMATION CONTAINED HEREIN.

This book is dedicated to my mom and dad,
who left the world too soon but were Spartans
through and through in their own way.

Many of life's failures are people who did not realize how close they were to success when they gave up.

— THOMAS EDISON

AUTHOR'S NOTE

Disclaimer: Living a Spartan lifestyle, although rewarding, can be dangerous and should be considered carefully.

CONTENTS

PROLOGUE:
THIRTY BELOW AND NOWHERE TO GO

THE RAID INTERNATIONAL Ukatak was an endurance race held in Quebec in the dead of winter, the absolute coldest time of the year. Temperatures are known to drop as low as thirty degrees below zero. Friends had talked me into doing this race — why else would I be standing at the starting line with three team members on a tiny island on the Saint Lawrence River in Quebec? To reach the finish line we would have to cover 350 desolate, barren, frozen miles. We would travel by iceboat, snowshoes, skis, and, believe it or not, mountain bike through nearly frozen rivers and snowy, rocky terrain that would discourage any sane person from entering. I knew this race was going to take six days if things went according to plan. I also knew that nothing ever went according to plan.

Despite the freezing temperatures, it was sunny and the sky was blue. The bright-colored gear of the competitors popped against the white snow. We began by iceboating along the Saint Lawrence River, which was like navigating a canoe seating four, with me in the back, through the Arctic Ocean. Floating chunks of white ice would knock into our boat and send us overboard, splashing into ice-cold water like seals going for a dip. But in a race like this, there was nowhere to go to change into dry clothes, nowhere to warm up. Once your clothes were soaked in ice water, your bones were chilled and would stay that way until the temperature rose. You were as cold as if you were naked. People die of hypothermia in these conditions. This was at the beginning of the race.

After we reached our destination along the Saint Lawrence, we hiked for two days straight through knee-deep snow in ten-to-thirty-degrees-below temperature. To muster the energy to keep going, I'd stop with my team when necessary to chug olive oil from a bottle. It seemed like logical choice to me: I could carry it, and it was loaded with lots of calories. In retrospect, it worked. But it wasn't without side effects.

Anyone who has done an ultraendurance event has at least some sense of the mentality it takes to distance oneself from one's body and keep pushing forward, impervious to every human impulse and basic common sense telling you to stop. Essentially your rational mind stops functioning, you lose the ability to reason, and you start functioning only in a primal way.

On the third night we trudged on snowshoes toward the top of a ridge, and images of my family members' and friends' faces appeared before me. Everywhere I looked, I saw their heads staring at me along the trail. For hours, I thought, What are they doing here? I also saw a McDonald's off the side of the trail . . . but it couldn't be, because I was in the middle of nowhere. Not only did the golden arches loom but the distinctive, pungent odor of a Quarter Pounder with Cheese and French fries blasted my nostrils. When you're starting to lose your mind like I was, it's amazing what grabs hold of it — in my case, apparently, trans fats and ketchup. I was officially losing it.

We were to rappel fifteen hundred feet down a cliff, at which point we would continue onward toward the finish line. We were in second place at this point, right behind the front-runners, still hopeful we could win — which was a shock for me, knowing I wasn't an athlete and had no business being here. The combined athletic experience of my teammates was measured in decades. I came from Wall Street, and before that, cleaned swimming pools. I would be relying on my mental toughness to make up for not being as physically fit as my teammates. This was the equivalent of the Olympics of adventure racing, and here I was, a pool cleaner, trying to keep up.

As we neared the ridge, I could tell something was wrong. The team in front of us had experienced a mishap: The ropes linking the ridge to the ground below had come loose and were no longer connected safely. To rappel down at that point might have ended with a red splatter in the pristine snow, a risk even we weren't willing to take.

There we were, standing at the cliff, with nowhere to go while the other team tried to figure out how to reconnect these ropes. We could hear commotion and saw headlamps lit below the cliff edge. When you're hallucinating human heads and golden arches, it's probably not the right time to be rappelling fifteen hundred feet, especially when the ropes are also having issues. With nightfall approaching, we saw no other way down, and we couldn't turn back now. The nearest camp, a few huddled tents, was the one we'd left at the beginning of the day. So, with the freezing wind swirling around us, we looked at each other without speaking, all thinking exactly the same thing: Fuuuuuuuuck. We would be spending the night in the snow without shelter, since bringing a fully functioning tent would have weighed too much to carry for six days. We hadn't planned on sleeping till we collapsed. That was our "plan." We had ignored the safety requirement of carrying a tent. Since we had no intention of using it, this would save weight.

This night was going to suck, but I didn't know how much. I burrowed into the freezing white because it was the only shelter from the Arctic blast of wind, but the conditions and the intensity of energy expenditure they provoked made it impossible to sleep. Those conditions hijack the rational part of your brain, the part of you that you think of as "you." All I could do was shake in misery until sunup, whenever that would come. I was in that state people must reach when they're lost in the wilderness, where they simply don't care anymore if they live or die, because if they die, at least the misery will come to end.

The next day, when the brief window of light appeared, we learned that the rope couldn't be fixed. The first-place team had made their way down, and we could either wait and hope they solved the problem or head out and try to catch them by foot back down the mountain. After discussing our predicament, we decided that we would try to ice-climb down this surface that you normally would only rappel. Every potential opening or possible path to slide, jump, or roll down that we evaluated had some fatal flaw, literally. This was like trying to hike down a triple black diamond ski slope that could never be skied. It was covered in waist-deep snow and littered with deathtraps in every direction.

Finally, we spotted one sliver of snow that seemed to work its way through the craggy rockface. Without much in the way of options, we began to climb down, searching for hand- and footholds. The ice was covered with snow and less stable than rock formations, but much safer considering our limited gear. This passage was so tight that we couldn't go far to the right or left or we might plunge to our death. We'd climb over fallen trees, and then suddenly we'd hit a ten-foot drop that would send us sliding precariously close to the rockface. This six-hour descent would be perilous at best. And I was just an average guy in an extraordinary situation. I had been training only six months for this event. I lived in New York City and had a desk job.

Finally, we made it to the bottom. I turned around, looked up, and saw the rock rising fifteen hundred feet up, except for this tiny little ribbon of snow area that we had come down. Looking up at it, we thought, Holy shit, how fucking stupid were we? A few feet in the wrong direction, and we would have been dead. Certainly an accomplishment, but not one I would ever repeat.

Later in the race, we encountered more difficulty. We were cross-country skiing for sixty miles, but because we had the wrong skis and no wax, we found ourselves in what seemed like a silly situation. We were on a cross-country ski trail where two small tracks exist for your skis. This tracked snow trail would go on for sixty-plus miles out in the middle of nowhere. The trail was very hilly with steep climbs and descents.

Pretty quickly, we realized we were stuck. Our skis could not get us up the climbs. We were skiing in place and not going anywhere. We looked at each other, frustrated, and popped off our skis — only to fall into waist-deep snow that was like quicksand. Although it sounds silly, we were literally stuck in our tracks. We couldn't go forward or backward, and when we had our skis off we couldn't get them back on.

Adrian, one of the guys on our team, had climbed Everest and was our resident expert. His presence had made me feel more comfortable about being out here in the first place; he was obviously a pro at handling difficult challenges. I looked at him like a nervous patient looking for reassurance from a doctor. At one point, he turned to me and said: "We got a serious situation here. This could be dire." That scared the shit out of me.

Yet somehow, we slogged through it, and eventually we caught a break when the temperature dropped. Apparently, for those who understand backcountry skiing — and we didn't — different waxes "stick" to snow at different temperatures. Like something out of a movie, and without notice, we were magically on our way again.

But that night I spent on the mountain hallucinating was the worst stretch of my life. I don't say that lightly, either; I've had some pretty close calls over the last forty years. Usually, when life presents such situations, there's a clear end in sight. Okay, maybe it's freezing cold out — but in two hours, I'll be back to the car, and I can crank up the heat. Sure, this procedure hurts like hell — but I can signal the doctor or dentist for more numbing agents if necessary. Yeah, I just stubbed my toe — but this too shall quickly pass.

That night, there was no end in sight. The sun would come up, but it would still be well below zero even in daylight. Under the best-case scenario, we were still totally screwed. No one was coming to rescue us. We still had to find our way down. And we did. Do that enough times, break through obstacles safely, and eventually you get this sense of security, whether false or not, that you're going to be all right if you just push through it. Let's face it, no matter what challenges confront me during my day, they probably won't be as severe as the circumstances on that ridge.

An inverse correlation links how miserable you feel in the race, and how great you feel after it, so you can bet I felt like a million bucks afterward. When you break through the other side of hell and finish an event that did not seem possible, that stopped you in your tracks over and over, something happens. You feel accomplished, incredibly proud of yourself and, in some ways, a different person.

Since the Ukatak, I have been lucky and stupid enough to compete in some of the most grueling endurance events in existence. When I tell people what I'm about to do, most of them look at me in a way that tells me they think I'm really stupid or suicidal. But you know what? There's a better way of looking at this. Challenging yourself to accomplish more than you know you can is never stupid — it helps show you what you are capable of. It creates a new frame of reference, one you can draw upon in the face of other things that are perceived as being tough in your life. It shows you possibilities you didn't know existed.

That's why I started the Spartan Race, and that's why I wrote this book.

SPARTAN UP!

1
FROM HERE TO INSANITY

Come what may, all bad fortune is to be conquered by endurance.

— VIRGIL

SPARTAN RACE WAIVER

All participants in Spartan Race competitions, races, or related events must understand, acknowledge, and agree that:

1) The risk of injury and death from participation in a Spartan Race or other event is significant. These risks include, but are not limited to: drowning, near-drowning, sprains, strains, fractures, injuries related to hot or cold temperatures, injuries from vehicles, contact with poisonous plants, animal bites, and stings.

In addition, injuries may result from accidents involving, but not limited to: paddling, climbing, biking, hiking, skiing, snowshoeing, travel by boat, truck, car, or other vehicular conveyance. All participants also acknowledge the risk of heart attack, permanent paralysis, and death. Spartan rules, equipment, and personal discipline may reduce these risks, but these precautions cannot exclude them entirely.

2) Acknowledging this fully, I knowingly and freely assume and accept all risks, both known and unknown.

This encapsulates the conditions all participants in my Spartan Races must agree to in order to compete. You may think I'm just covering my ass, but if you think about it, this is also a pretty good waiver that everyone should sign just to participate in life. I know because this is how I live my life: The Spartan Way. I can tell you that the rewards far outweigh the risks.

My name is Joe De Sena and I grew up poor in Queens, New York. I was never much of a natural athlete, but nonetheless athleticism would eventually become my calling card. You see, I am the founder of Spartan Race, which has gone, in the span of ten years, from a crazy obstacle race in a field to a multimillion-dollar global lifestyle company. A million hard-core fanatics now define their world around the code that we have created for them, and many more participate. Every weekend thousands of people flock to our events, which are staged year-round across the globe. They are looking to better themselves, hoping to "Spartan Up!" and all that phrase embodies and means. And I am their biggest supporter and their worst nightmare — often at the same time.

People may think I'm crazy, sadistic, relentless, maniacal, suicidal, all rolled into one, but they still seek me out, sensing somehow that there is a method to this madness. And that my tactics change lives, create opportunities, and yield results.

In 2009, Noel Thompson, one of the U.S. Olympic wrestling coaches, sent his wrestling team to train with me for a weekend. I had met Noel at one of my races the prior year and he was intrigued by my unique and sometimes crazy training methods. He thought I could help his team.

So the day they touched down at Rutland Airport after a five-hour flight, I made sure that they were confronted with the unexpected. They were not told why they were coming to see me, and they didn't know what they would be experiencing upon arrival. Their coach had arranged the trip, but some of the best wrestlers in the world were in the dark about the venture and what kind of training they would encounter.

I wanted to give them a proper introduction to the Spartan

lifestyle, so I had a driver pick them up at the airport and then un-ceremoniously drop them off on the side of the road—Route 100 in Nowheresville, Vermont. My farm, which doubles as the Spartan Race world headquarters, was their destination, a mere ten-mile hike over a series of hills and turns with very little shoulder. It was freezing cold, and they tried to make a few calls, but they were in the middle of nowhere and out of cell phone range. Dressed for a business meeting rather than a mountain hike, they had to walk the entire distance carrying their luggage. So off they trudged to train for the weekend with some lunatic in the mountains far away from their state-of-the-art wrestling gym.

To the team members, this seemed like insanity, or at the very least rude. This was not how Olympic athletes were treated. Yet, there was a method at work. These were some of the best wrestlers in the world, but like most of us, they had been guided their whole lives, in this case by their coaches. I needed to see how they would react when their mettle was tested in a crazy fashion. Great wines come from overstressing grapes, diamonds come from coal placed under enormous pressure, and a sword requires intense amounts of heat and a lot of forceful pounding before it becomes an elite weapon. Likewise, how these wrestlers responded to the stress of my training protocols would determine if they were not only Olym-pic-quality athletes—I already knew that much—but if they were champions. After all, there is only one gold medal for each weight class.

For their training, I had them chop an enormous amount of wood in the rain and the carry and stack it. They did a ton of hik-ing. I have a giant spool of wire that's about five feet in diameter and weighs probably three hundred pounds, and I had them roll that up a mountain. It was muddy, so there was a constant risk of them slipping and this wire ball rolling back over them. They car-ried sandbags up and down the mountain, they dug trenches, they rock climbed, they swam — they must have swum eight miles. They did a lot of Bikram yoga in 110-degree heat.

They were not happy at first — it was not the training they had prepared for over the last fifteen years, and it made no sense to them. They grumbled among themselves and wondered aloud what they were doing there. They were only there because their coach had made them go.

It made no sense, that is, until months later, when I received a call from one of the wrestlers. He had just won the world championships, and he wanted to thank me. His frame of reference had shifted while he trained with me. Now, you're on the mat and you've got ten seconds left, your opponent's beating you, and you're like — I did forty-eight hours straight with that lunatic in Vermont. I can get through the next ten seconds. That was the difference between him being a world champion and not.

The obstacle race where I had met Coach Thompson months earlier had required a stretch of kayaking, and at one point, competitors were forced to drag their kayaks twenty yards through waist-deep mud and weeds. All the other teams made it through, but Noel, who was trailing his team by one hundred yards or so, got stuck. Not in the mud, mind you; his mind vapor-locked, preventing him from even wading into the muck with his kayak as all the other racers had. I instinctively grabbed him and his kayak and pulled them both through the mud. On the other side, I was able to push them downriver.

He, like so many others I have seen, could not adjust to a foreign situation. He had avoided mud his whole life, and once he sank into it, all those fears and all that programming — from parents, from teachers, you name it —"Don't get dirty!"— suddenly bubbled to the surface and paralyzed him. He had no idea how to deal with this obstacle.

Later, after the race, Coach Thompson approached me. "Can I talk to you?"

"Sure," I said. "What's up?"

He said, "How did you learn to do that?"

"You just get in the mud and go." I hadn't thought twice. That's how I always tackle life: put one foot in front of the other, focus on the little goal right in front of you, and almost anything is possible. As a result, I have learned to push through when others stop, even this coach who trained world-class athletes. How could he freeze up during the race? In my mind, you just commit to something and then get it done, no matter what. He had let self-doubt creep in — a major mistake I see people making all the time.

You won't get stuck in mud during a wrestling match, at least not during Olympic wrestling, but you might get stuck in a crazy hold or some other predicament. Wrestling is among the most fluid of sports. An Olympic match has a beginning and ending, but how it unfolds during those five minutes is anybody's guess. There's no telling how much energy you'll need to expend or what you'll encounter. Wrestling isn't linear like a marathon. Your opponent may be wholly unpredictable, continuously trying to place you in unexpected holds from which you can't escape.

So Coach Thompson sent his wrestlers to me because he knew that I could help them prepare for the unexpected. I could teach these elite athletes that if they endured enough off the mat, they could crush any challenge on the mat. My goal wasn't to help them prepare to win; it was to help prepare them for the unknown.

No physical element embodies the unknown like mud. It sticks to us, slowing us down, trying to pull us under. Since the beginning of humankind, men and women have been forced to deal with this brown muck. Mud delayed Napoleon at Waterloo, crippled the Nazi invasion of Russia, and turned the Ho Chi Minh Trail into an obstacle course for insurgents in Vietnam. That mixture of earth and water that gets caked on your shoes has changed history. I'm guessing it's slowed you down a few times as well.

In a Spartan Race we always confront competitors with mud puddles and swamps, things you only run through out of necessity. These obstacles help condition them for "the mud" of everyday life, the stuff that drags us down, or at least tries to. Maybe you didn't get that promotion, but we teach you to persevere in your job anyway. Maybe you got dumped, but we still want you to seek a new partner with a positive attitude. When you're already fatigued and struggling, the addition of mud can make for a toxic mix, exacerbating the desire to surrender. So every course has at least one mud trap somewhere along the way. It wouldn't be a Spartan Race without one.

But that's only the beginning. A Spartan Race wants you to achieve more. That's why we put a brutal and unforgettable course in front of you. Our mission is to wow our racers, push their minds and bodies to the limit, and help make them healthier through superior, extreme, and challenging obstacle races. That is why Spartan events are designed to challenge people to overcome breakdown.

My goal with every Spartan Race is to push you to overcome your short-term desire for comfort in an effort to reach for something greater than your current self. Anyone can run up a hill. What about going up the same hill crawling under three hundred feet of barbed wire? Obstacles and mental challenges force our athletes to be agile and capable in movements that are lateral as well as linear, and to be resilient in the face of plenty of surprises.

Spartan Race is for anyone and everyone looking to make a difference in their own life and in the lives of those around them. The typical path is this: Start with a Spartan Sprint, a three-mile race with fifteen obstacles; work your way up to a Spartan Super, which is an eight-mile race with twenty obstacles; and then set your sights on the biggest, baddest of all the Spartan events, the Beast, a 13.2-mile event with twenty-five obstacles. Those lengths were not chosen arbitrarily. I determined that the Spartan Sprint distance should be based on what people in today's society are able to do: anyone should be able to jump off the couch and complete three to four miles. The Super would be challenging but still accessible to reasonably fit, first-time competitors and for athletes accomplished in other sports. The Beast was designed to test the will of even the most hardened athletes.

Our season ends in September with the Spartan World Championships, so many of our racers come out of hibernation after the holidays and start building up their endurance in January. This cycle repeats itself every year, only with many more participants every racing season.

This isn't a sport where the founder and co-owner (that would be me) watches the games unfold from a cushy air-conditioned box, waiting for a five-second TV cameo after a fumble or touchdown, the camera checking to see if I'm pissed or celebrating with my fancy friends. At Spartan Race, we all throw ourselves into the fray, and I hope to interact with, or at least acknowledge, everyone who races. No matter where I go, the question most frequently asked of me is "How do you stay motivated?" That tells me that the thousands of people asking me that question do, in fact, need our help staying motivated. It's not easy, but it's worth it.

Most Spartan racers are well along the path to getting motivated, but others are just getting started. To me, our races engender a greater sense of purpose than what's produced from marathons or other traditional endurance events. I think it's because Spartan Races are so challenging on so many levels; yet at the same time, they're very accessible. The person floundering in a dead-end job isn't going to tackle an Ironman. But they just might pony up eighty dollars to enter our three-mile Spartan Sprint.

You'd need to attend one of our races to appreciate their uniqueness and energy. They feel and sound like a sporting event and a rock concert rolled into one. We're the New York City Marathon meets Burning Man, with some other primitive craziness thrown in for good measure. Were you to attend the race, you very well might ask yourself, "Who *are* these folks walking around covered in mud and drenched with sweat, chanting in unison at the start of the race? Where did they come from and what compelled them to do this voluntarily? It looks really freakin' hard." The level of dedication from our racers is reflected in our completion rates. In the early days, it was 65 percent, and now it's probably closer to 90 percent, although that number drops a bit when it comes to a Beast. One by one they will tell you something like:

"I was fat."

"I was out of shape."

"I was bored with my life."

Then they found Spartan and everything changed.

Spartan racers are a fairly representative cross section of American life. Age-wise, the bell curve would be a bit steeper — you won't see babies crawling in the mud, and our courses would be too tough for all but the most-stout senior citizens, although we would encourage them if they wanted to try. For the most part, you'll see men and women from their teens through their fifties tackling the course at varying speeds. These aren't just super athletes, although many of them are indeed. We're talking super moms, cancer survivors, the weight-loss crowd, and others with fierce determination.

Likewise, you'll find that the occupations of the Spartan racers reflect mainstream America. Our races attract investment bankers, students, active military members, schoolteachers, plumbers, police officers, and firefighters, among many other professions. Some racers come from other sports and fitness realms such as marathons, triathlons, bodybuilding, CrossFit, mixed martial arts, and yoga. For still others, this is their first dive into any organized fitness activity.

Why do people go to such great lengths to participate? Why would people subject themselves to that sort of undertaking with no tangible benefit awaiting them, other than maybe a T-shirt and a pat on the back? Why do I, and others like me, run these incredibly demanding races, taking on courses that could destroy us and, at a minimum, make us feel helpless at times? Didn't we invent cars, air conditioning, and elevators precisely so we wouldn't have to endure stuff like this?

From small spinning studios to dance classes to CrossFit "boxes," there is definitely a movement toward fitness afoot. Spartan racers subject themselves to a hellish test of will and physical strength rather than sleeping in on a Saturday morning. They do this because they want something more out of life than comfort, mediocrity, and a fancy toilet bowl brush. They likely sensed, without necessarily articulating it, that preparing for such a race and then running it would make them better — even if, at the moment, most of them looked like they were at war.

The Death Race

The roots of Spartan Race lie in a different sort of war, and one image encapsulates it more than any other for me. In 2005 two former marines — 4 percent body fat, six-footers, ripped — lay in the dirt crying next to a woman who was removing one of her legs. She proceeded to dump water out of it, and then she methodically put it back on, as if this were an act she performed every day. If you happened on this scene, you might think you had stumbled into hell or onto a movie set, only the tears were real, and the prosthesis was not a prop. Never mind the fact that few movie scenes are this strange.

But this was reality. These people were competing in an event called the Death Race, a brand-new kind of race my friends and I had invented to either break competitors or inspire them. This was well before the concept of Spartan Race had come into existence, but the seeds of an extreme sport that could appeal to the masses were being planted along the trails of those Death Races all along.

Earlier that morning, I had told these three competitors that they needed to swim three miles in icy water. They made it, but their times weren't fast enough, according to the rules I had established—rules of which they had just been informed. While they could continue along the course, they were no longer official competitors. The woman, an amputee, adapted and immediately continued under the revised terms. Even though I knew she was disappointed, she shrugged it off without a second thought. But the ex-marines simply could not accept this change in the program; they could not adjust their frame of reference. These men had served their country with honor and were model citizens in every respect. You might even call them heroes. But they were throwing temper tantrums in front of me, a far cry from the behavior expected from battle-tested men.

But the Death Race will do that to an otherwise accomplished and well-adjusted athlete. It's meant to push the envelope, meant to take competitors to the edge—and beyond. A brutal forty-eight-hour test of mental and physical endurance, the Death Race is as much an exorcism as it is a footrace. Our no-frills website for the event, youmaydie.com, offers competitors this guidance:

> This is the ultimate challenge. The Death Race is designed to present you with the totally unexpected, and the totally insane! This endurance race is comprised of mud runs, obstacle racing, trail racing, physical challenges and mental challenges all in a +48 hour adventure race. 90% of you will not complete this

endurance race. Please only consider this adventure style race if you have lived a full life to date.

We hold three Death Races a year. We have a summer Death Race, a traveling Death Race, and a Team Death Race. Each Death Race has a theme. One year it was religion, and the race started and ended in a church. For the year of betrayal, we planted cheaters on the course for others to follow. The Death Race described above was gambler themed, meaning participants rolled the dice in hopes of cheating death. In many Death Races, competitors run for up to fifty miles over the dark green mountains of my hometown of Pittsfield, Vermont, population 546. Over the course of a year, more people come to Pittsfield to face death than actually live in the town.

The Death Race goes for as long as it takes to only have 15 percent of the participants remaining; the race "ends" when 85 percent have quit. Until then it is game on. This creates two enemies in the eyes of each competitor: their fellow competitors and us, the organizers. What makes the Death Race truly unique are the obstacles and challenges along the way. Some of these obstacles serve a specific purpose; some we come up with just to mess with people. The head games begin long before the race itself. Without explanation, competitors might be asked to bring a tuxedo, five pounds of hay, a life jacket, five dollars in quarters, and a pound of grass seed to the race. The goal is always to raise the stakes of the unexpected.

Once the race starts, challenges might include diving for pennies, eating onions, extracting stumps from the ground, carrying kayaks and tires for an ultradistance, lifting rocks for six hours, chopping wood for five hours, completing three thousand burpees — anything to try to make people quit. There's a method to this peculiar brand of madness, though. I believe that confronting these insane obstacles is the best way to rewire a human brain after years or even decades of coddling, predictability, and excuses.

At the race that included the two marines, the last organized cutoff known to the racers was the second night before at our property at Riverside Farm. It's always a good feeling to have every "good" racer pass through the checkpoint, and to know which racers have decided to quit. I love when we can account for everyone, especially when it's so late in the event.

Day three starts to get a bit dicey, though. The competitors are exhausted and the support staff is shot, too. It happens when you put people in such extreme conditions with so little sleep, but especially so with the folks racing, who are missing that chip that tells them to slow down, or stop, or quit. Some people aren't wired to respond to the cues from their body; they're wired to complete their goal. At any cost. In some ways this is risky, but in other ways it's encouraging people to get in touch with a more primal survival instinct or mechanism. It's incredible to watch them compete, and you're never entirely sure what's going to happen.

On the final night, we told the racers to come to White Barn at Riverside Farm at 6:00 A.M. sharp the next morning, dressed in a tuxedo with their required gear and backpacks on, ready to continue the race. We surprised them when they arrived with a mock casino setup. They were invited in one at a time to play a game of poker. When they got to the table, I offered them a choice: They could take their "bib"—proof that they finished the race—or they could go for it all, which would earn them the coveted skull we purchased for $13 from CVS. It was a major gamble: If they decided to go for the skull, and then lost, they would lose their bib and go home completely empty-handed, with no proof that they even competed. It would be as if they had never finished the race. Why do this? People gamble every day with their lives, relationships, health, and so on. The race forced participants to begin thinking in those terms of how they gambled each day.

I have incredible respect for these individuals; they had suffered so much already, only to be denied their reward, and now they were lining up to complete a new challenge, even though they were totally physically beaten and barely awake. But it was a final challenge and the only way they were going to get their skull.

Three hundred and fifty participants had started the race, and at the end of this final gambling challenge, twenty of the folks who were skull-less still felt they deserved them. This happens each year: A percentage always feels as though it was unfair, just like life. Even if we agreed with them, we had only seven skulls left to award. After huddling up and brainstorming, we had a solution: We told them the race was going to go back to the place they went yesterday, Blood Route, a terrible hike eighteen miles away in rugged mountain dirt roads, a challenge that was ridiculous even by Death Race standards. We assumed at that point the twenty complaining of their unfair results would say no thank you and go home. Instead, things got ugly. Husbands were kissing their wives goodbye, grown men were falling over and crying at the thought of going back out there, and I didn't blame them one bit. I would have started crying at the prospect too.

Yet here they were at the crack of dawn, lining up again. One of them unable to put on shoes was duct-taping his feet as a possible ridiculous solution to his issues. My offer of redemption meant going back out there to finish what they couldn't do quickly enough the day before and do it on what was becoming an oppressively hot day. I really couldn't believe it — *they were going to go.* Only, we had lied. We were going to make it a sprint to the finish without telling them; a few miles from the white barn, we would stop the first seven to arrive, award them, and tell the remaining thirteen we were sorry they missed the cutoff. We had laid out a three-mile route with race coordinators located at every mile. Their instructions were to give the racers ten minutes to complete each mile. If they didn't reach the checkpoint in time, they were done and stopped, even if coordinators literally had to pull them off the course. End of story: Only the seven fastest through the checkpoints would call themselves finishers.

It didn't make sense but it made sense to us. Changing the rules and misdirecting competitors is part of the race. These people who lined up were going to sprint three miles at most, and the first seven would be crowned victors and receive their skull trophy. That was it. The race would be over. I'd be at the river with the kids by lunchtime. How could this go wrong?

My wife, Courtney, took the first checkpoint by our covered bridge, a half mile from the starting line. She would be telling racers who were trailing that they were done and could go home. Some people were really running, an amazing sight to behold. Some were dragging their bandaged zombie bodies and looking for a way to get out of this terrible ordeal. One man actually had duct-taped his shoes back together — the race terrain had wreaked havoc on his fancy two-hundred-dollar sneakers. Still he was moving really quickly despite his appearance.

I will never forget one guy who barely made the cutoff. I had been counting down, and he made it by a few seconds after my Courtney yelled, "Keep going!" That guy deserved to stay in the race. But I had to end the race for everyone after him. "Turn back and get your families," she said. "Get some sleep, see you next year." A few people did turn back, but others refused to stop. They came right at her, their zombie-like stares boring through her like she wasn't even standing there. They were not quitting. There were several "I'm sorry, ma'am, but I'm not stopping" comments as they bumped past her.

"It was an awful feeling," she said. "I saw the look they gave me and I saw their switch was turned *on*. I've seen that look in Joe so many times before. It's the place he goes when he's just decided in his head that he's going to keep going and that nothing — not his tired body, extreme temperature, or a stronger opposition — will keep him from getting to the finish line."

Those guys kept going and broke through her checkpoint. Her first thought was: *Why didn't they believe me?* And then: *Where the hell are they going?* She used her loud angry mom voice and was as stern as she's ever been. But they still ignored her. Then it dawned on her that they thought the finish line was eighteen miles away through some brutal terrain, and that's where they were heading. Holy crap, she thought — there's no way this could be backfiring so badly. She couldn't believe that they were willing to go there, to push on, to beat up their body more than seventy hours into the race. They were like bacteria that had gotten too strong for our antibiotics. They got into their "zones" and would not stop.

She called ahead to the next checkpoint and explained to two other staffers that these guys were on a mission. They were a runaway train heading for the last official race checkpoint before the trailhead opens up into the national forest where they were heading. Once the racers passed that checkpoint, it was actually going to get dangerous. No water, no checkpoint, no volunteers. The last man standing between them and danger was Andy Weinberg, the race director. Andy is incredibly charismatic and speaks the language of the supercrazy ultraendurance athlete because he is one. Andy told Courtney not to worry. "Go to bed. The race is over."

Not exactly. The final seven skulls had been awarded to the "official finishers," the guys who had run the fastest. Standing in front of the entrance to the national forest, Andy was able to convince many of the Death Racers that the race was over. Except, that is, for five men who refused to stop and went rogue. They acknowledged the race was over but continued to go on anyway, knowing full well that they were on their own. They had decided that they were going to go on no matter what, and they were completing a mission in their own Death Race brain, which, at the moment, was not functioning properly.

This was now a dangerous situation. These five were all trained military guys, and given that it was summer, they probably wouldn't die from exposure. But losing racers in a national forest is not great publicity. I feel that a competitor in a Death Race should be prepared to break an ankle on a poor ax swing, or suffer a laceration or hypothermia or even a heart attack — those are all legitimate risks that racers assume. But actually losing someone is just not acceptable.

Even though racers sign a waiver saying "You may die," they are still our guests. They are great people with compelling, inspiring backstories. The have lives, families, responsibilities, and I care about all of them. So after looking at the facts and weighing the risks, we decided to go after them.

Two of the support staffers followed after them into the national forest on Blood Route. Courtney, Andy, and I would drive thirty miles or so around the mountain on the main roads, hoping to see them if they emerged from the forest. I'd had the most sleep and Courtney was lecturing me the whole ride, so about ten miles in, I hopped out and headed down a path. Andy and my wife kept driving.

Assuming the competitors had continued on the correct trail and the travels had gone perfectly, it was still a dodgy plan. But it was all we had. Courtney was upset and freaked out by the thought of losing one of these guys. She was also furious with herself for not getting the competitors to stop at the first checkpoint. We had our whole crew out there looking for them, and we were exhausted too. It was a bad scenario. We hadn't planned for these guys to leave the reservation. In the nearly ten years that we'd been putting on races, nothing like this had ever happened. Based on how slow they were going and how dog-ass tired they were, we felt like we might be out there looking for these guys for a long, long time.

Late in the day, rainy and cold, we finally spotted them — the marines — sitting on the edge of the lake. They were hungry, thirsty, tired, and hallucinating. We had talked about what we would say if and when we found them; how to make them stop; how to convince them that they were off course, that the race was over. But Courtney was so relieved and yet angry to see them that her mom instincts came bubbling up and the whole intervention strategy went out the window. She jumped out of the car and ran right up to them, to their visible disappointment. They probably thought Andy or I would be the ones to yell at them or give them some award for being the "most crazy." One guy later told me he thought there would be confetti at the finish line, near the lake. What?!

She explained that they were off course and the race was over and it was time to get in her car and drive home. She told them that a wilderness search party was looking for them — which was true — and that it was time to call it quits. No one budged. Having seen this vacant look in my eyes before, knowing how high the stakes were and that it was her last chance to avert disaster, Courtney — normally the sweetest person you could possibly meet — lost it: "Get in my car *now*!" she screamed. "My husband and my friends are out there looking for you selfish assholes, and you're messing with your lives now!" On and on she went, screaming at and shaming them because it seemed like the only way to convince them that this race was truly over.

They all walked to my car except the guy with no shoes and duct tape wrapped around his feet. He said he didn't care what I did or said. He said that he had survived cancer and now he was running to honor children stricken with the disease to show them that they could defeat the disease and go on to accomplish great things in life. He also was competing to raise money that they needed so badly for treatment. He couldn't go on physically, but he couldn't give up mentally, either.

Said Courtney: "Well, then, I'm your shadow. I'm going with you. I hope you know wilderness survival skills because you're going to need them to save me later tonight. You are now stuck with me." She was in flip flops, jean shorts, and a tank top and not prepared for any hike, let alone an eighteen-mile death march back to Pittsfield.

At that point, the guy started getting emotional. Finally, he climbed into the car with the other guys. They all fell into a fitful sleep. Courtney drove around until she finally found me and the members of the other search party, and we all rode back. The competitors were totally shot yet undoubtedly they would have gone on, limping and trudging through the dirt roads and the mud and the mountains just because they loved pushing themselves and finding their edge and what they could really endure, creating new boundaries for themselves in the process.

When people hear me say "You need to suffer" in reference to the Death Race and the training that goes into preparing for one, I don't mean that you have to be miserable. I mean that you have to challenge your expectations and leave your comfort zone. When you push your body to its limits, when you are out of breath and in pain, when you are lying on the ground exhausted — that's the kind of experience that reveals to you how bad things could be. By doing this, you're changing your mind's frame of reference to a new set of standards. When that challenging workout is over, the small worries of the day seem like nothing.

The Search for Modern-Day Spartans

The Death Race was the precursor to the Spartan Race, a more structured version of that ultra death-defying event. But Spartan

Race is based on all the same principles. You see, the Death Race is, in fact, a carefully orchestrated effort to find a certain kind of person. The kind of person who might seem driven and type A in "normal" life, but who could put those qualities to maximum use in certain environments and situations. "How many of these people exist in the world?" I asked myself. Most people disappoint, and, in our society, 99 percent of folks are looking for the easy way out. But that 1 percent — what do those people have that the rest of the world doesn't? As it turns out, along with being tough and gritty as hell, they have an ability to delay their gratification and constantly change their frame of reference, two concepts I'll elaborate on as the book unfolds.

After three to four hours in the Death Race, everyone is already exhausted; the rest of the seventy-plus hours is pure grit, meaning the resolve to complete the race even when every fiber of your being wants to quit. People in the Death Race aren't looking for fame or recognition. They do it in pursuit of personal goals. Grit is doing something unpleasant or painful over an extended period of time. People in the Death Race are actively pressing on. They signed up, and with each passing hour they're choosing to endure the pain even as it intensifies.

Physiologically, what you're doing is resetting your body's set point for stress. Our fight-or-flight mechanism is supposed to kick in when we are running from a lion to save our lives, not when our brussels sprouts are slightly undercooked, and not when we are worried that our house isn't as big as that of a former classmate who we just reconnected with on Facebook. The easiest way to convince your body that sitting in traffic is not worthy of a stress-induced freakout is by showing your body what real stress feels like, in the controlled setting of your daily workout.

Every morning, I always make sure I get my sixty minutes of pain — it releases all types of post-hard-work pleasure chemicals and the rest of my day feels easy in comparison. Periodically, I need to take it a step further — I have to push the absolute limits of my body. I need to go on a ten-hour bike ride or a middle-of-the-night hike with Andy. I know I have successfully reset my frame of reference when I collapse on the concrete and it feels better than a Tempur-Pedic mattress.

Whatever situations may come up during the rest of my day, they won't be stressful in comparison. If I was able to push through that last set of burpees when my muscles were all shaking, that last quarter mile when my lungs were on fire, then I can easily handle whatever obstacles come up during my day.

In a marathon or triathlon, you know exactly what's coming. In the Death Race, you don't know the obstacles and challenges in advance. This pays dividends long after the race ends. People often leave a Death Race with a crazy sense of purpose. I think it's even more so than with marathons or other traditional endurance events, because it's so challenging on so many levels.

"This race was a game changer for me," said Will Bowden, a first-time Death Race competitor and fifth-place male finisher in 2013. "Any situation that brings you to your mental or physical boundaries, or both, and allows you to decide if you want to hold short or cross them and create a new boundary, will always change the core of your being. The Death Race did just that."

Many people have come up to me and said, "Your race changed my life, Joe." And the reason is because it builds what we call "obstacle immunity"— the ability to overcome unforeseen obstacles without becoming excessively stressed. In scientific terms, it is the ability to avoid the fight-or-flight response to a situation, to remain calm and able to think clearly. This quality is borne of the kind of preparation that prevents the individual from getting stressed out by unfamiliar obstacles. Here are a few classic example of obstacle immunity put into practice, spanning thousands of years:

1. The Stoics of ancient Greece believed that the greatest obstacle was not death, not pain, not suffering, but cowardice. By training themselves to accept what they could not change and to be courageous in front of any obstacle, they eliminated their fear of death.

2. Tibetan monks identified the lack of control over the mind as the greatest obstacle. So the monks spend days making sand mandala paintings, and when they're done, they sweep away their work with a broom. It's not about the destination; it's about the journey and the process that gives them the opportunity to practice awareness, focus, and control.

3. Kung fu students have to overcome the obstacle of fatigue. So the master has his students carry railroad ties to the top of the mountain and then carry them back down the mountain. There is no productive accomplishment, but the student will no longer find it challenging to run up the mountain carrying only his own body weight.

4. Michael Phelps's coach Bob Bowman identified the greatest obstacle as unknown challenges that might cause his athlete to lose focus. So Bowman prepared Phelps for the Olympics by picking him up late before a meet, so he'd have to skip a meal; or by breaking his goggles before practice, so that they'd fill up with water while he swam. When Phelps's goggles broke during the 2012 Olympics, he was able to push through it to win gold.

No matter what dreams a person has, athletic or not, they will encounter obstacles along the way. When you ask people what they want out of life, you get very different answers. The perfect life for a thirty-year-old man on the streets of Thailand means something different than the perfect life for a sixteen-year-old on a sailboat in the Hamptons. It's doubtful whether there is any ideal "good life." At some point in life we will all encounter pain and disappointment.

A relative will die unexpectedly. A friend will betray us. We will lose money. Shit happens, as they say.

So Death Race is kind of rough, right? It's a little scary. Yet you commit, and then you persevere, and somehow you survive. And everything else in life is kind of insignificant. You were wearing a nice suit or dress to work and it rained. Not a big deal. Or your coffee is too cold, or your car didn't start in the morning, or the kids are screaming. All not a big deal anymore, because you've built obstacle immunity. You start to feel a lot better about yourself. You've got some confidence. It becomes contagious. It's a life-changing event.

In any given Death Race you'll find elite athletes, Olympians, Navy SEALs, Division I football players, wrestlers, and other physical specimens. No matter what they've done in other realms of life, we inspire them to reach a new level. Afterward, the e-mails are usually some twist on the same refrain: "You changed my life. This was unbelievable." It's not like they won the lottery with us and we gave them forty million dollars. It's not like we all of a sudden gave them a beautiful wife. It's not like we all of a sudden gave them great children. All we did was give them a taste of what it once was like to be a human being.

We receive something in return: inspiration. "We started the Death Race to find people that we'd like to hang out with," explains Andy. "We wanted to surround ourselves with people who inspire us. The people who inspire us the most are those who don't waver, don't quit, don't take shortcuts, and don't fall short. Each of us can be one of those people if we choose to be. Sacrifice time now for more time later."

The Spartan Starting Line

Due to its extreme nature, Death Race is open only to elite athletes who have the time to train extensively. But there was a huge majority of the population who were missing out. So we decided to create a more accessible version of that event, one that would bring the exhaustion and exhilaration of extreme, adventure, and endurance racing to a million or more people who otherwise would never have experienced it. Spartan Race would include elements of the Death Race, yet it needed to be standardized and developed into a sport people could realistically participate in, one that would appeal to both first-time athletes and serious competitors. Only in doing so could we create a mainstream fitness movement and change the world for the better.

The initial concept was hazy at best, except that it would be a footrace through natural and man-made obstacles to test competitors' physical and mental fitness. It would incorporate dry land, water features, mud, and even fire. Ultimately the entire race design was really determined by whether a given obstacle or challenge was something a human should know how to do, should be proficient at, had been doing in some form for millennia. In short, everything on the course should be functional, requiring no special equipment — just a lot of heart and the DNA that makes you want to survive and thrive.

At first we didn't know what to call this new race. I remember sitting in the kitchen of our farmhouse with Andy, Courtney, and other associates, rattling through dozens of names. They all fell short. The name had to say it all, it had to give a visceral feeling when said in public, and it had to be serious.

I thought back to one of my high school history classes, where we had learned about the Spartans from ancient Greece. The stories about these warriors resonated with me then and had stayed with me ever since.

"Let's call it Spartan Race," I said.

Everyone fell silent. There were no dissenting opinions, no need for debate. That was going to be our name because the Spartans seemed to personify everything we stood for and everything we conspired against. They were strong, brave, resourceful citizens with no tolerance for bullshit. They were known far and wide for their ability to defeat much larger populations and military forces through force of will. They focused on mind and body in equal measure.

We also liked that they dated back to antiquity, since so much of our philosophy rebelled against modern society while hearkening back to simpler times when you could venture out into the woods without a GPS system to guide you, blaze your own trail rather than looking for the other guys' shortcuts, and start your day without a coffee from Starbucks. Andy would say, "Having a tough day? Imagine what it was like in Thermopylae."

Organizing this sport, enterprise, or whatever you want to call it became consuming. I begged old friends from Queens, I begged family members, I begged anyone I met to help us expand this idea of an easier, more formally structured Death Race. Something that anyone could compete in. Something that could become an Olympic event. We started telling whoever would listen: "Just sign up. Don't worry about whether you are in good enough shape."

We found that the minute people signed up for a Spartan Race, they started training harder. They were motivated to complete the course, so all of a sudden they started pushing themselves to exhaustion during their daily workouts. It's normal to train really hard before an event, so they did. And when they got to the event, they were in the kind of shape they had hoped they would be, and they were able to cross the finish line along with everyone else. They also found themselves finding more fit-minded friends.

You might think this is all crazy . . . but imagine if everyone started doing this.

2

CONFRONTING THE GREATEST OBSTACLE: YOUR WILL

You run the first half with your legs, the second half with your mind.

— OLD RUNNING PROVERB

I HAD JUST DROPPED ten feet out of the window and hit the concrete. It gave my eleven-year-old body a jolt, and now I had to get to my bicycle without anyone seeing me. I was running away from home and heading to my grandmother's house twenty-five miles away. To get there, I would navigate a major New York parkway with no bike lanes or cross bridges, figuring out where to turn and which direction to go on the fly. In hindsight, it was a sign of things to come.

I was born in Brooklyn and grew up in Jamaica, Queens, in the 1970s and '80s, an unlikely setting for a modern-day Spartan to rise from the ranks. My dad was a serial businessman, and it didn't matter the industry, whether it was pizza parlors or airfreight. He made good money, at least for a while, and doing so involved him working hours so long that I don't remember him ever not working like crazy. It didn't matter whether we were at home or on vacation — he was working very close to nonstop. It was a trait of his that I would inherit, although it wouldn't manifest itself until later in life.

This helped us to live comfortably, which was great. But his addiction to working nonstop came with a price, and even comfort has its downsides. I remember being a cocky little kid thinking, "I don't need to go to college; I could just work with my dad!" I would complain about things that I wanted or that weren't "perfect" in my life. Truth be told, I was a spoiled brat.

Beneath the surface of normalcy lay a dysfunctional family life. My father was Italian and we lived in an Italian neighborhood reminiscent of the movie *GoodFellas*. My parents would have fistfights in the house, and my mother was hospitalized more than once with injuries as serious as a broken nose. Many of my family members went to jail, and a few haven't been let out. My parents and grandparents used to tell me they were in the military when we went to visit family in jail to protect me from the truth. Later when I learned the truth, it also came with a neighborhood adage: "You have to be able to do the time . . ." Whenever I'm in pain or just wanting something to end, I think, It could be worse.

One way my dad tried to make up for all of his excesses and broken parenting skills was to offer us quick fixes in the form of treats and permissions. He'd say, "Let's have Chinese food," and, "You can stay up late." It was his attempt to make up for all the crazy shit that was going on. Of course, as kids, the treats and the freedom to hang out at night fueled our childhood imagination.

My mother was the yin to my father's yang. Whereas my father was focused 100 percent on business and making money, my mother was focused 100 percent on health and wellness. When I was three years old, her mother died from cancer, a disease that struck at much higher than normal rates in the section of Queens where we grew up, maybe because we lived near a garbage dump. This loss sent my mother, aunts, and uncles in search of answers. Eventually it led them to a newly opened health-food store in the middle of our Queens neighborhood. Why a store like this popped up in a district of sausages, pasta, pizza, clams, mussels, and wine is beyond me, but it did.

The man who worked there changed my family's life forever. Swami Bua was a tiny but powerful Indian yogi with wispy white hair and forked feet who had moved from India to New York City to teach and practice yoga and meditation. Talk about an endurance monster: He could blow into his conch shell, Louis Armstrong style, for many, many hours on one single breath. He had known everyone from Mohandas Gandhi and Bertrand Russell to Muhammad Ali. When he died, some folks said he had been the oldest man on earth.

Inspired by this remarkable man, my mother did yoga, ate healthy food, and meditated. She instilled this same love of healthy living in me, drilling all sorts of important lessons into my head at every turn. Chief among them was that life was not worth living unless you lived it to the fullest. My mother was a delayed gratification expert without even knowing it. My mother had it right, only I wouldn't appreciate that until later.

In the late 1980s, when the stock market crashed and real estate values plummeted, my father's financial fortunes tumbled along with them. My parents got divorced and I moved with my mom and my sister to Ithaca, New York. My father was supposed to pay my mother's rent as part of the divorce settlement, but his own business was collapsing, and that meant, more often than not, that he couldn't help us. We rented a small house and couldn't afford to keep rent payments up, or pay heat bills, or own a television set.

That day I fell out of the window and headed off to my grandmother's house? It was actually my *father's* mother's house where I sought refuge. My mother was the disciplinarian in the family, and once my parents divorced and my father no longer lived with us, my mother became even more strict, sometimes hitting me with a wooden spoon or other utensil as I became more and more difficult. That day I left, my mother had been all over me, screaming and just doing what a strict mother does.

So I wanted to go live with my grandmother on my father's side, who was even easier and more lenient than he was. She gave us anything we wanted, and I could watch TV and eat junk food all day. Funny in retrospect, I turned out to have a complete distaste for a lack of discipline in life, because as a child, I gravitated toward it, like many kids do.

Truth be told, being flat broke is not as bad as it sounds. It makes for a simple life and simple wants. I found myself just wanting to make sure that we ate, that I could work out, that I could save for college tuition, and that we weren't thrown out of the house. This was tough for a formerly spoiled kid with a once-rich dad, but as with everything in life, you make it through or you don't. And when you emerge from the struggles, almost every other development in your life seems like good news in comparison.

In retrospect, this downward financial spiral was the best thing that could have happened to me, because it totally recalibrated my frame of reference. It made me appreciate many of the things I was used to and was bored with earlier in life. I was happy with much less, so anything above that baseline meant much more.

Ultimately, these experiences, as unpleasant as they were at the time, helped make me the man I am today. I said to myself, "I'm never going to be in a situation where I go to start a family and I don't have money." I made a vow never to be miserable and abusive. I would work to crush my goals and rise beyond all expectations to be an exceptional person. To this day, you never see us "abusing" the Spartan racers. We are training, teaching, and being hard on them to make them appreciate what they have and to become better human beings. That is the soul of Spartan Race.

So my plan became to work crazy hard, sacrifice in the present to make money, and not get married until I had money and I was removed from the insanity I had witnessed as a child. I thought, "I'm going to spend the next fifteen years working hard while my friends are partying." I would crush my goals by outworking and outhustling the next guy, undeterred by any obstacle that might appear before me.

Part of that was deciding that I wanted to attend Cornell, an Ivy League school, even though I was not a naturally gifted student by any means, and I didn't even really know how to study. My buddy at the time was like, "Hey, I'm going to party all summer because we have to buckle down this fall." I said, "Fuck that, I'm going to study all summer so I know how to study when I get into school." He ultimately went to University of Las Vegas, while I got into Cornell. I have approached almost everything in my life this way by getting "ahead" of the project at hand, whether it's doing my homework in advance or training for a race.

To make money, I started cleaning the pool of our next-door neighbor. I didn't know it at the time, but he was the head of the Bonanno organized crime family. I thought he was just a great neighbor interested in helping the kid next door earn a few bucks. The opening of that single door changed my life forever. I ended up cleaning or building pools for anyone and everyone involved with the "five families of organized crime" that either had a pool or wanted one built. It became a multimillion-dollar business with a clientele of seven hundred customers, a lucrative and well-oiled machine that employed family and friends and paid my bills and then some.

During my twelve years running the business, I was in top shape because I was doing very physical work seven days a week. As a result, I could eat whatever I wanted to without gaining weight. However, by the time I reached Wall Street, I was still eating that way, so I packed on some pounds. Soon enough, I was really out of shape.

What happens to recent moms or athletes or anyone eating to support a lot of physical labor is that their body keeps eating that way when they are no longer as active. A body in motion tends to stay in motion. My mother used to say it's easy to exercise if you're exercising.

A year or two later, I got roped into something that sounded ridiculous by a friend who was on the cover of *Men's Health* magazine and had the perfect physique. He wanted me to do an adventure race with his team. Sure, I had been feeling like I really needed to try to get back into the shape I was in when I was hauling pool equipment day and night, but to the uninitiated this race sounded insane. Still, he was relentless and he finally got me to the starting line. Looking back on it, this event changed my life. I discovered a truth that would guide much of my life thereafter: when you sign up for something, you're forced to train for it. Just like in a business: you're forced to work. Just like having a kid: you're forced to take care of it. All of a sudden, you become accountable.

My first endurance event was a half marathon, which I entered cold, without training or other preparation. The feeling was like what a drug addict must feel like after their first hit — I was hooked. Something had been triggered in my brain. I was a kid who had felt helpless against tremendous forces and forced to run away. Now I was running *into* something, transcending the very limits of fear, uncertainty, and my own body. I had diligently earned millions from the pool biz, but that hadn't been enough. Now I was facing the demons of my being and beating them. That supercharged me.

For my fix, I took up obstacle and adventure races. I started with a three-hour adventure race of biking, swimming, kayaking, and running and loved the kaleidoscope of challenges it presented. Who wouldn't love feeling like an Olympian or a Navy SEAL? An explorer? We were out there doing stuff that I had only seen in the movies. I was an adventurer, and it felt incredible. Getting back in shape was child's play compared to the effect endurance events had on me. They were helping me define who I was and who I needed to become. I started waking up super early, eating super healthy, and finally following my mother's wisdom on yoga, which she had tried to impart to me for twenty-five years. I also started to find friends who enjoyed these unrelenting challenges as well.

I kept raising the bar after every race. I'd ask everyone I met in the field: "What's harder? What's harder?" "Give me the hardest thing you got" became my mantra. I became addicted to backing myself up against the wall. The crazier the race, the more I wanted to do it. My perseverance hardened during races that others would call crazy.

In 2001, I did the following events:

- Raid International Ukatak, Canada, January
- IditaSport: Alaska, February
- Odyssey Adventure Race, Big Island, Virginia, March
- OAR Beast of the East, Clayton Lakes, Virginia, April
- Raid the North Extreme, Newfoundland, June
- Adrenaline Rush, Dublin, Ireland, July
- Discovery Channel World Championships, Saint Moritz, Switzerland, August

The harder the race, the more I loved it. I imagine it's almost what an astronaut feels — experiences so alien from daily life that returning to "normal" becomes very hard, because normal now seems so unsatisfying. My endurance résumé filled up with more than fifty ultraevents, including twelve Ironman events in one year alone. Most of my races have been one hundred miles or more, with a few traditional marathons thrown into the mix. Once, I did the Vermont 100, the Lake Placid Ironman, and the Badwater Ultra all in one week.

Nothing, though, was as difficult as doing the Iditarod on foot, which is crazy. It was thirty degrees below during the whole race.

Yet I kept trudging forward for ten days. Imagine peeing on yourself because the thought of pulling down your pants is even worse. Imagine falling into water so frigid that your limbs immediately go numb. Imagine your eyelashes being frozen shut — yet hallucinating that bears are chasing you. Oh, and did I mention that you're starving?

I was out of my mind and, at times, out of my body. Whether I was running toward or from something, I willingly put myself through hell, forcing myself into situations where water, shelter, and food preoccupied my every thought. At those moments, everything else that I thought was important in life, all the things I had stressed over for so many years, vanished. My determination to push my body to the edge became a parallel effort to understand what drives folks like me.

The Second Half of the Run

An old running proverb goes, "You run the first half with your legs, the second half with your mind." Believe it or not, you can make it eight days beyond the moment when you think, "I can't take another step." I like to tell people to take no money and run in one direction as far as they can, so that they have to run back home. That's Spartan-like behavior. This book, and the Spartan Race, is really about the second half of the run, when your mind cannot only play tricks on you but also compel you to quit or will you forward. Yet distance is a relative concept. A long run for you might not be long for me or the next guy or girl, and vice versa.

Humans have remarkable resiliency that often goes untapped, but in fact, history is dotted with incredible feats of endurance, insane tests of will that seem almost impossible. I not only attempt similar feats, I study them. I consider their genesis, analyze how they unfolded, and do postmortems on where and how they went off the rails. Sometimes the smallest overlooked detail can bring an enterprise to the brink of failure. To me, these expeditions are a metaphor for life as it should be lived. These men and women were willing to stare down death to fully live.

Sir Edmund Percival Hillary did something that no man had ever done before when he and a fellow explorer, Tenzing Norgay, reached the summit of Mount Everest in 1953. They were part of a Royal Geographic Society expedition, one that included a dozen climbers, thirty-five guides, and eighteen tons of gear and food. That's the sort of massive support it took to get two men within striking distance of the peak, via a particularly treacherous route.

One team had already failed to reach the summit when Hillary and Norgay made their attempt. Hillary awoke that morning to find his boots frozen solid and stuck in the ground. He had to wait two hours to start the final ascent because that's how long it took him to get his boots out of the ice before trekking the final short distance. Undeterred, they pressed forward, and at 11:30 A.M. on May 29, 1953, they reached the top of a mountain that soars to 29,035 feet. Hillary declined to be photographed by Norgay on Everest's summit. Hillary was a true Spartan: he wouldn't grandstand, even while on top of the world.

This wasn't his only noteworthy accomplishment. Hillary also reached both of the Earth's poles and devoted much of his life to helping the Sherpa people of Nepal. He would later lose his wife and daughter in a plane crash in the Himalayas, and he barely missed the flight that ended up colliding with another plane over Queens, New York, in 1960. Our Everest-like highs in life are fleeting, if we are lucky enough to achieve them at all. They are a time for reverence and humility, not fist pumps and chest bumps.

In another of my favorite Spartan-worthy adventures, a man named Steven Callahan spent seventy-six days adrift on an inflatable raft in the Atlantic Ocean after his boat sank. Somehow he had the presence of mind to dive down and retrieve some essential supplies from the submerged boat. Over the course of eighteen hundred nautical miles, he survived on the mahi-mahi and triggerfish that he speared. He rigged up tools to capture rain for drinking water. He even managed to maintain a regular exercise regimen during the voyage, even as he lost one third of his body weight. On Callahan's seventy-sixth day at sea, fishermen picked him up off the coast of Guadeloupe. He later wrote a best-selling book, *Adrift*, chronicling his ordeal.

This sounds like a hellish experience, and in many ways, undoubtedly it was. Imagine the stress of circling sharks, hunger, thirst, loneliness, malfunctioning equipment, and rescue near misses — Callahan saw nine ships, but the crews didn't see him. He had salvaged a harpoon gun after the shipwreck, and at one point he missed the fish he was aiming at and punctured a hole in his raft. Imagine boredom verging on insanity, yet potential dangers as far as your eye can see. Imagine taking the most uncomfortable moment of your life, exaggerating it tenfold, and enduring it for seventy-six days straight. Yet Callahan also achieved transcendence during this epic voyage, describing it in his memoir as "a view of heaven from a seat in hell."

These stories of endurance and eventually triumph in the face of great adversity inform the Spartan story. As in the case of Callahan's time lost at sea, it's not always simply a physical challenge. Callahan was at the mercy of the ocean for that entire journey. What made that journey so indelible was the perseverance and ingenuity it took to survive.

In many ways, this is what differentiates Spartan Races from other sports and activities. Sure, it takes endurance and physical strength to surmount the obstacles, but that's not nearly enough; you must also figure out solutions to crazy, unexpected problems along the way, all while keeping your wits about you. If Callahan had been in incredible shape with a chiseled physique, it would have helped him — but only up to a point. The real key was having the wherewithal to retrieve those supplies after the shipwreck, to build rain-capture devices, to fish with no fishing rod . . . to survive.

Then, take the survival tale of Swedish adventurer Göran Kropp. In October 1995, he left Stockholm, Sweden, on a bicycle and rode it to the base of Mount Everest, arriving there in April 1996. He climbed Everest, reaching the summit with no oxygen mask and no help from Sherpas. He descended the mountain and eventually pedaled back to Sweden. If someone invited you to undertake such a wild adventure, you might say: "That's impossible!" or "You're crazy!" As it turns out, it's not impossible. It's hard — *really* hard — but doable under the right circumstances. The cliché is true: where there's a will, there's a way. Seemingly insurmountable challenges confronting you in business, sports, health and fitness, and relationships are far more manageable than you might imagine.

The last two expeditions I want to mention weren't a single feat, like climbing Everest, or an accident, like Callahan's disaster at sea. These were meticulously planned expeditions of discovery, one focused on the American West, the other on Antarctica. First is the Lewis and Clark expedition, familiar to many of you from your school days. Commissioned by then-president Thomas Jefferson after the Louisiana Purchase, this was the first major expedition to explore and map the United States beyond the Mississippi River. Captain Meriwether Lewis, Second Lieutenant William Clark, and a group of other men began in Saint Louis, Missouri, and made their way by canoe through Missouri, Nebraska, and the Great Plains and ended up at the Pacific Ocean in Oregon before retracing their route home. They left in May 1804 and returned home in September 1806.

Remarkably, given that it was a two-and-a-half-year journey, the only casualty was a sergeant who died as a result of appendicitis.

But when the explorers set out to explore new territories, their rudimentary maps were lacking, leading to problems at every turn. An account in Jefferson's library of an earlier trip west had suggested to Lewis and Clark that they somehow could carry canoes from the Missouri River to the Columbia River. Unfortunately, the Rocky Mountains were in the way. That was only one of many challenges surmounted by these brave and adventurous explorers. Winters were devastatingly harsh, food scarce, and native populations often hostile toward these interlopers from the east.

Lewis and Clark made historic contributions, from the 140 maps they drew to the more than 200 plants and animals and more than 70 native tribes they discovered. None of it would have happened if they and their men hadn't personified the Spartan mentality. These were not men who grew up driving to the supermarket in air-conditioned cars to purchase factory-manufactured foods. Today we think of doing an Ironman as a phenomenal accomplishment: 2.4-mile swim, 112-mile bike ride, and 26-mile run. Or a marathon: people train six months to run one, and when they cross the finish line, it's the coolest thing they've ever done. Well, Lewis and Clark did that pretty much every day for twenty-eight months.

In other words, everything is relative. By the time I did my first Ironman, I had already completed eight ten-day races, so the Ironman felt like a warm-up to me. It took "only" twelve hours. I thought, This is unbelievable. This is easy. In contrast, if the most strenuous thing I had ever done was walking to and from the supermarket a quarter of a mile away, an Ironman would have posed an unbelievably imposing obstacle. I was not a natural athlete by any stretch, and I never thought I could do an Ironman when I first heard of one. But after doing these multiday adventure races, I knew I could. It all depends on your frame of reference.

With those experiences under your belt, real problems don't

seem overwhelming. Without that experience, we end up with adults exclaiming, "Oh, my God! The kids are screaming. The bag of groceries broke. What a horrible day! Today is a disaster." Disaster? We have no idea what a real disaster is. Many people feel unnecessarily entitled to things they have no business feeling entitled to, like fancy cars and consumer electronics and other luxuries. It's unfortunate, but that's how our society has evolved.

Imagine life 150 years ago. A bear chased you in the morning while you were trying to get wood to heat your home. A fox ate your chicken. Now you must fix the fence so it doesn't happen again. Oh, wait, your son develops pneumonia so you have to hike eighty miles to get medicine. It sounds hard, but I think everybody needs to suffer a little. The threshold for pain, the tolerance for obstacles, used to be so much higher than it is today. We try to re-create those obstacles from those days gone out on our Spartan Race courses.

When you read the journals from Lewis, Clark, and their men, they don't talk about being depressed, despite their extreme hardships. They were too busy trying to stay alive to mope around. Yet today, depression is rampant in our society, including among the well-to-do. All this material wealth hasn't made them happy.

No adventure resonates with Spartans more than the Imperial Trans-Antarctic Expedition undertaken by Sir Ernest Shackleton and his crew in October 1914. If the Spartan Race has a patron saint, Shackleton is that man. Shackleton accomplished some amazing things during his life and was knighted along the way, but one of his feats stands out above them all as the embodiment of Spartan-ness.

Twice, Shackleton tried unsuccessfully to become the first man to reach the South Pole. Unfortunately for him, in 1911, a Norwegian explorer beat him there. Losing such a prize could crush a man's soul. People remember guys who arrive first and plant their flag. The guy who arrives second is easily forgotten. Can you name the explorer who reached the New World after Christopher Columbus? Even with the lunar landing, three men arrived at the same time, but we remember Neil Armstrong, the first man to plant a foot.

Still drawn to Antarctica despite, or perhaps because of, his disappointment, Shackleton, at age forty, conceived of his own consolation prize: he would aim to become the first man to cross the frozen continent end to end through the South Pole. He would need two crews of twenty-eight men (including himself), one each for two ships. One ship would drop him and his team on one side of Antarctica, while a support crew would head to the other side of the continent. Those men would station supplies along what would be Shackleton's team's homestretch and then pick the men up if all went according to plan.

No one could accuse Shackleton of false advertising, given that his ad read:

<u>MEN WANTED</u>

FOR HAZARDOUS JOURNEY. SMALL WAGES, BITTER COLD, LONG MONTHS OF COMPLETE DARKNESS, CONSTANT DANGER, SAFE RETURN DOUBTFUL. HONOUR AND RECOGNITION <u>IN CASE OF SUCCESS</u>.

ERNEST SHACKLETON

Five thousand men responded, and fifty-six were chosen. Sixty-nine Canadian sled dogs would also join the expedition, a decision that would prove lifesaving in ways that even Shackleton likely didn't foresee.

After sailing south from Buenos Aires for six weeks, Shackleton's ship, the *Endurance*, came within one hundred miles of land when the ship ground to a halt. It was surrounded by pack ice, which floats along the ocean's surface, turning it into a giant ice tray. The weather wouldn't be warm enough to thaw the ice until spring, still many months away. No one else knew the ship's location or predicament, and outside help couldn't have reached these stranded mariners anyway. No one else in their right mind would be crazy enough to travel there even if they could.

After ten months, the shifting ice crushed the ship. The men abandoned it at Shackleton's command. They set up camp on a giant ice raft with only a fraction of their original provisions and only three of the four original lifeboats. Subsistence meant hunting penguins and seals in nearly constant darkness. Shackleton tried to lead several marches off the ice, each time needing to cover hundreds of miles to be successful, and each time failing. This left the men in a more exposed, vulnerable position than before, but with even fewer amenities. The dogs were ultimately shot and eaten so the men wouldn't starve to death.

The giant ice slab had floated some thirteen hundred miles when it began to melt; one dire circumstance now gave way to another. The men would need to cram themselves into the three rafts and attempt to drift to the Elephant Islands 150 miles away, with survival by no means assured. They made it, but the islands weren't much more hospitable than the sheet of ice they had just escaped.

Realizing that they were beyond the reach of any sea lanes or trade routes, Shackleton settled on a last-ditch effort to survive: he and several of his men would attempt to make it 850 miles by sea to South Georgia Island, a voyage through frigid waters that would require an almost miraculous feat of navigation. Somehow they made it — only to find that their landing spot was on the wrong side of the island. So they had to march thirty-six hours across mountains and glaciers.

Shackleton ultimately saved all of his men, but he died on his ship en route to another polar expedition when he was forty-eight years old.

What these men — adventurers, pioneers, survivors — held in

common was that they each reached a point where they had no real choices left. Hillary wasn't going to be denied immortality just because his boot was frozen into the ground. Callahan had to turn his raft into a floating ecosystem to survive at sea. Lewis and Clark couldn't turn around just because their maps were inaccurate. In Shackleton's case, he realized that he and his men could eat the dogs, or they would starve to death; that they could make that dangerous sea voyage, or they were going to die miserable deaths on that godforsaken island; that they must hike across South Georgia Island without resting for even ten minutes, because had they fallen asleep in that cold, they never would have awakened.

None of these were easy calls. But Shackleton's resonates the most with me because on the one hand, it was a feat of pure endurance; but on the other hand, it was incredible project management.

Finding My Own Way Home

We may not have mapped new territories or been lost at sea, but Andy Weinberg and I raced all over the world. Wherever we'd go, I'd ask, "Could I live here?" I was seeking an escape from shortcuts, gadgets, and all the innovations designed to make life easier and safer. I wanted to get back to the way things used to be. I was in another country doing an eight-day race when it hit me. The local villagers we encountered everywhere we went were always smiling. They always seemed happy. They had everything they needed because they lived simple lives. It started to make more and more sense. That was for me, and that's what I wanted for my family, too.

That place turned out to be Pittsfield, Vermont. So in 2003, I took some of the money I had made on Wall Street and purchased an organic farm sitting on 140 acres. After I moved my family to Pittsfield, we quickly became entrenched in the local landscape. I became a family man working the land using organic gardening methods. I yearned for simplicity, and I had time to focus on what lay ahead: working the soil and raising my kids.

When we landed in Vermont, it was a tough few years. Locals didn't accept us right away, there was no traffic, not even the good kind, and everything shut down during hunting season. People had different priorities and news traveled fast. It took some time, but ultimately, it turned out exactly as planned — well, sort of.

Pittsfield, Vermont, was supposed to be my retirement home. Some retirement. Other members of my inner circle not only visited my new digs, they started moving there, too. There are probably ten of us in all up there now. It took some convincing when Andy told his wife he wanted them to move there. "My wife is from Kansas City, Missouri, a big metropolitan area with about five hundred thousand people," he recalls. "A Bed Bath & Beyond seemingly on every other block, concrete everywhere, highways with six lanes. So I moved her to Vermont, and she calls herself a pilgrim, whereas in my case, the outdoors is what I love. Now my kids are being raised in a place where it's safe, it's clean, people are happy, and there's a lot going on. For us it's much better, and now she enjoys it. She likes the simple life."

Am I intense? Yes, and I'll be the first to admit it. I completed more than ten thousand burpees a few weeks ago because our new marketing team roped me into it. I have an enormous passion for life, as does the whole Spartan team. When you are someone with that kind of passion, I feel like you owe it to the world to share it. What drives it? I'm sure at some level it's a response to my troubled relationship with my father. It's okay to respond to emotional pain from childhood with positive addictions and a keen sense of self-improvement. As adults we are too often paralyzed by such antiquated anguish, and we find ourselves repeating the same mistakes hundreds of times because we are ruminating over that which we have no power.

Instead, I turned my pain into an outboard motor and learned how to steer the boat to happiness and success. The pain will never really go away, but I have trained it every bit as potently as I have trained my body.

I have had this recurring dream my whole life. In it, I'm stuck. I'm trying to move faster but I can't. Running but not being able to get away — a poignant reminder of the moment I leaped out that window.

I have been building businesses since I was a kid, and every day, from the second I wake up and light hits my face, I know what's got to be done. It's like the old saying: if I don't do it, then who will? I have been reflecting lately that this passion needs to be shared because everyone should have it toward the things they want to accomplish in life.

Spartan Up! Life Lesson No. 1: Every Obstacle Presents an Opportunity

In ancient times, a king had a boulder placed on a roadway. Then he hid himself and watched to see if anyone would remove the huge rock. Some of the king's wealthiest merchants and courtiers came by and simply walked around it. Many loudly blamed the king for not keeping the roads clear, but none did anything about removing the stone.

Then a peasant came along carrying a load of vegetables. Upon approaching the boulder, he laid down his burden and tried to move the stone to the side of the road. After much pushing and straining, he finally succeeded. After the peasant picked up his load of vegetables, he noticed a purse in the road where the boulder had been. The purse contained many gold coins, as well as a note from the king indicating that the gold was for the person who removed the boulder from the roadway. The peasant learned what many of us never understand: every obstacle presents an opportunity to improve our condition.

— Author Unknown

3
OVERCOMING OBSTACLES, TOSSING YOUR COOKIES

When you are going through hell, keep going.
— WINSTON CHURCHILL

SO YOU'VE SLOGGED through the mud and scrambled out of a ditch. Great. Ready for a pat on the back? Wait, that's a twelve-foot wall before you. And you must climb it. Only it's been greased, so that just when you reach for the top, you might fall backward eleven and a half feet and land on your ass. Then you will have to try it again, and again, and again, each failure reinforcing the one before until you finally make it over the top. "C'mon, Joe, are you serious? Did you really have to grease the wall — isn't it hard enough as is?"

"Spartan up!" The title of this book is a phrase I bark at people every day in one situation or another. Those two words have a simple meaning: stop complaining and get it done! "Spartan up!" is an attitude, an X factor, a way of life that I would sum up like this: Challenges make me tougher. Failure makes me work harder. Knock me down, and, sure as shit, I'm getting right back up.

To me, the ancient Spartans extolled a fuller and deeper sense of values than we understand and appreciate today. Honor, valor, courage — these were the things held up as marks of a life lived well. Honorably. They worked as a team, every man living for every other man, defending his brother to make sure that everyone else around him was safe. There was this unique and inviolable bond among these men. And nobody was tougher.

These ideals are reflected in the relentless training that began when Spartan youth were pulled from their home at age six or seven and turned over for military training that became their reason for being thereafter. At age twelve, the intensity of their training skyrocketed. By age twenty, they were ready for enlistment in the Spartan army, assuming they measured up. Those who did were now warriors and members of the premier fighting force in the world.

They weren't sitting there with guns. They weren't sitting there firing off missiles. They were *in it*. Consider the armor they needed to carry and march with and fight with, sometimes for days at a time. If you had to pick up that armor, you'd be struggling to hold it after five minutes.

When I think of the Spartans, I also think of camaraderie, or some combination of loyalty and teamwork that was even more intense than that. Love them or hate them, there was nothing like being part of the Spartan brotherhood. They exemplified excellence. You won't excel at anything until you put in the work, and the Spartans were more determined than anyone. They were lionhearted, every single one of them. That was *required* from all of them in order to be part of that team, so when they were there, they knew it, and they loved it.

At the same time, Spartans behaved the way they did because they were responding to a horrible adversity. There was a dark side to their society, because they were essentially culling their own herd (tossing infants with defects, fighting their own weak to death) in order to make themselves strong enough to defend and protect their resources.

If that was all there was to them, they would have been barbarians. The code of honor they lived by, their camaraderie, the respect they had for their women, their honor in battle — these qualities redeemed them and made them people worth emulating.

I could have reacted to the abuse I experienced as a child by becoming a bully. Instead I became an athlete with the honor and endurance of a Spartan soldier. And we all can do that! To become a Spartan in your own life is to become both fearless and relentless. That's the goal here, whether you're fighting an army or tackling a problem at work or school. We use the obstacle race as our foundation because we're trying to transform lives, and life itself is an obstacle course.

Physical barriers, career challenges, injuries, viruses, addictions, bad luck, self-doubt — countless obstacles may appear in our path at some point during our life. They don't always do us the favor of coming one at a time, either; often, one obstacle seems to beget more of them, until it feels as if the entire universe is suddenly conspiring against us. It's often a divorce that comes around the time you get laid off that corresponds with a health problem that accompanies a crazy neighbor moving in next door, and so on.

In life, the biggest obstacle, the tallest wall, can be imaginary. It can exist only in your mind. Some people stay stuck to one spot for years because they are paralyzed by the fear of change. They may be stuck on the couch. They may be stuck in a dead-end relationship. They may be stuck in a lousy career. They are stuck in a prison of their own design.

We've been conditioned to think that we as a society should spend tremendous resources eliminating obstacles from our lives, rather than teaching people how to surmount them. "Easy" is the greatest marketing hook of all time. Six-pack abs? Easy, buy this gizmo. Great physique? Easy, take this pill. Want people to notice you? Easy, plastic surgery.

Unfortunately, the effect these so-called solutions have on

obstacles is the opposite of their intent. When the most difficult obstacle that you encounter in everyday life is finding the will to get up off the couch and walk to the fridge, then that is the level of difficulty you are prepared to survive. When you are confronted with the life-equivalent of a twelve-foot greased wall (getting laid off, getting divorced, losing a loved one), you'll be squashed like a bug on a windshield.

The enormous spike in divorces in recent decades, as well as the rise of single hyper-indulgent and hyper-protective parents and "helicopter" two-parent households, has voided at least two generations of children of the "rite of passage." Without rituals of endurance, transcendence of nature, physical tests, and the mysteries and rites of man- and womanhood, we are becoming far more cerebral, insulated, and fearful of the outside world. Physicality has become alien rather than second nature. Spartan Race provides people with a rite of passage, and this is why the response to it is so often life-changing, spiritual, and even metaphysical.

Easy has never been my way of doing things. I'm not a naturally gifted athlete or thinker; I just gut things out until I'm successful. I know there are easier ways to get things done, but persistence always wins. I wasn't the best high school student. I didn't see the point of hitting the books hard, and it wasn't my priority. Then, six months before I graduated high school, one of my classmates said to me, "Why don't we go to Cornell, since it's in Ithaca, near where your mom lives?"

I saw this idea as a new challenge, and it fueled my imagination. This kid's dad was a professor at Cornell, so we quickly applied. Thankfully, they turned me down. Thankful? Yes, I was thankful rather than upset because I love the word *no*. Those are my two favorite letters in the English alphabet, in fact. This rejection only made me even more determined to go.

So I did my research, and I found a loophole in the system: I could take classes there without being formally accepted as a student. So I attended classes, applying and reapplying for admission all the while. Three times they rejected me, until finally they accepted me. Since each semester as a non-student I could only take a limited number of credits, my last semester I had to take twenty-eight credits, or nine courses. It was a nightmare, but I had learned how to study by then. One of my professors shared with me a technique for whipping material into my long-term memory. Every night I came home and I wrote out all of my class notes. The process was laborious, but it worked. I didn't even have to study for exams anymore.

I had met an obstacle and figured out how to move past it. It wasn't easy, and it took me a while, but I did it. And having conquered that obstacle, I felt better prepared for any future obstacle I might encounter in my life.

If you know obstacles are coming, how do you prepare for them? One of the key tenets of the Spartan Race is that we fill our course with obstacles that deliberately seek to trip people up. Essentially, you're practicing encountering the unexpected. It sounds paradoxical, but it's not. Special forces like the Navy SEALs and Green Berets train this way all the time. Combat is the ultimate example of encountering unpredictable situations, and those who excel in such situations have trained themselves to be ready for anything that comes their way. Special ops are so intriguing for just that reason — they are cool under pressure, all business under even the most extreme circumstances. This is an extremely attractive trait that many of us admire.

For thousands of years, induction and training in the military was itself a rite of passage for young men (and often young women) around the world. So it's not so much the militarism of Spartan Race that I'm alluding to, but the fact that Spartan Race fills a niche that military training and the rituals and social mores that went along with it used to fill. Not all of us will or should experience combat, but this unpredictability is one reason why we advocate training outside in nature as opposed to inside a gym. Running up and down hills with variations in weather and terrain is different than running on a treadmill in a climate-controlled room.

Consider the example of Sarah Marbach, who as a twenty-one-year-old college student weighed 440 pounds. She had settled into a routine whereby she would go to class, come home, and eat, and then go work, come home, and eat. Doctors told the twenty-one-year-old that she wouldn't make it to thirty if she didn't change her ways.

Her mother had undergone gastric bypass surgery, and she encouraged Sarah to consider the procedure. Sarah finally attended a health seminar on this medical procedure. Gradually, her dire health circumstances and the death sentence they represented sunk in. "I knew this was going to be the tool that I would need to save my life," she recalls.

During the latter half of 2009, Sarah changed her lifestyle in anticipation of surgery, cutting back on her calories, increasing her workout frequency. By the time she was wheeled into the operating room, she weighed in at 330 pounds, 110 fewer than she weighed at the seminar. Post-op, she continued her healthy ways. She arranged her schedule around her favorite exercise classes: spinning, kickboxing, and Zumba. She ate in response to hunger, not boredom. She hired a personal trainer to guide her through her weight-training sessions.

Sarah decided to attempt a running race, something that would have been unthinkable when she weighed 440. She studied her options and began running. She completed 5Ks, a few 10Ks and then a half marathon. At this point, her body weight was normal for her height. "I began to feel great about myself and my achievements," she recalls.

Then she heard about the Spartan Race. "I was eager to take on the challenge but a little intimidated," she says. "When I heard *The Biggest Loser* sponsored a team that competed in a scaled-down version of the Spartan Beast, I jumped at the chance to be a part of it."

The moment of truth came on June 1, 2013, when Sarah stood at the starting line with her fellow *Biggest Loser* team members. The race started with a mountain, and Sarah covered the incline at a trot. Every time she started to fade, her father's words of encouragement would push her forward, or one of her teammates would chime in: "Get it, girl! This is all you!"

Then came the obstacles. "They were all challenging in their own way," she says. "Yet I was eager and willing to try every single one presented, even if failure meant taking my penalty burpees. I focused on what I was able to complete and didn't beat myself up about the burpees. I climbed up walls ranging in height from six to eight feet, ran through tires, carried a sandbag up a mountain and back down the other side, dragged a concrete block up a mountain and back down again, dragged a huge tire, climbed a wall made out of ropes and a slanted wall, and crawled through mud and under barbed wire."

While working her way through a mountain pass, she heard a voice behind her. "You don't know how much you just inspired me!" one of her teammates barked. "Just knowing that I was able to inspire a fellow racer because I wasn't going to take the easy way out is an amazing feeling," she says. "That's really been a theme in my life, and the Spartan Race was no exception."

The help worked both ways: many a Spartan helped push Sarah over walls to help her continue. She failed to complete the rock wall, the pegs, the rope climb, the spear throw, and the monkey bars. She was forced to do thirty burpees each time. Rather than viewing these setbacks as defeats, she now viewed them as areas to improve upon for her next Spartan Race.

In the Spartan world, we recognize that the key to success is commitment. The best way to get committed is to take the first step toward whatever it is you're doing. When I start pedaling from Vermont to see my family in Long Island, I'm committed. Halfway there, I'm exhausted, my muscles hurt, but I have no choice but to keep pedaling. Once you sign up for a Spartan Race, once you tell all of your friends about it, you, too, are committed. To back out is to admit failure not only to yourself but also to others. This should motivate you to honor your commitment and show up at the starting line ready to race.

Each obstacle in the Spartan Race hits the human body in a different way. Here are a few examples of key obstacles that you'll find in most Spartan Races and the physical attribute they test:

Monkey bars: upper-body strength
Log walk: balance
Rolling hills: cardiovascular fitness
Spear throw: hand-eye coordination
Cinder block drag: endurance

The beauty of obstacle racing is that it exposes your weakest link. You might be great at marathons but lack upper-body strength. You might be strong but lack the endurance needed to climb hills. No matter how well prepared you are to meet life's challenges, one weak link can do you in. You might be great at making money but lacking in relationship skills. You might be strong enough to overcome physical illness but struggling to overcome emotional guilt. Obstacle race training is designed to give you the confidence to attack your weaknesses. You used to stare at the rope climb and wonder how in the hell you were ever going to do it. But you tried, and you kept trying, and now you own that rope. If you can overcome that obstacle, then you can learn how to overcome an addiction, bad habits, inertia, unhappiness, anything that is dragging you down.

No matter what form an obstacle takes in life, it usually isn't supposed to be there. When I would run ultraendurance races, I'd be going along and *boom* — a shift in the weather, a landform that wasn't supposed to be there, something totally unexpected that I hadn't trained for. I learned that you *can* train for this unpredictability. We assert that you can develop a mindset that allows your instincts to take over when something appears in front of you from out of the blue. Once trained, your mind isn't clouded by the confusion wrought by the unexpected. Instead, the unexpected obstacle sharpens your focus. You can process the new data and adjust on the fly to new circumstances.

The twelve-foot greased wall embodies numerous physical challenges in one event. Climbing a wall when you're already tired and beat is hard enough, but it becomes way harder when the wall has been greased. Your grip gives way, your feet start moving frantically to keep you moving up, and the slightest hesitation can send you stumbling back to earth. For a Spartan, the first response to a challenge is not a question of can or cannot — it's a question of do or do not. And for the Spartan it's always do, no matter what. And if she can't beat the obstacle, she trains until she can.

Our racers run not only to complete the event but also for a time, one that can be compared with those of other competitors or with past times. I would argue that the biggest obstacle of all becomes time. A Spartan or Spartan hopeful must forge a new relationship with the concept of time. Every minute on this planet is precious. We're only allotted a finite number, and we don't know in advance what that number is. For that reason, I consider time management to be a reflection of one's character. Are we getting our work done or slacking off? Are we disciplining our kids or spoiling them? Are we buying health food or processed junk?

Tossing Your Cookies

Most decisions in your everyday life will not be life and death. The challenge for all of us today is that we have all sorts of options, most of them designed to make things easier at every turn. Devices to make life more convenient, offers that allow us to renege on personal commitments, pills to help us stay awake, pills to put us to sleep, "workouts" where you hold a shaking piece of metal — shortcuts galore. Spartans don't look for shortcuts; we take the harder route because that is the path that offers the greatest reward. We delay our gratification, even if that gratification holds no guarantee.

Remember Shackleton's ad: "HONOUR AND RECOGNITION IN CASE OF SUCCESS." Their sacrifice guaranteed nothing. It gave them only a chance at glory.

This is always a tough sell. People don't naturally take pain first in exchange for the hope of pleasure later. People naturally seek pleasure on top of pleasure, which is how two out of every three adults in the country wind up overweight or obese. Too many people lead sedentary lives, and chronic diseases such as type 2 diabetes are skyrocketing as a result. Eighty-three percent of these illnesses could be avoided through better diet, exercise, and smoking cessation. I would go so far as to say that the number one form of medicine is exercise.

The quick reward, the prize right before your eyes, holds powerful allure. Most everyone takes the easy route. The hard route is the one less traveled. Those men Shackleton recruited could have stayed home in their warm beds with their wives, but they chose to delay their gratification. Delayed gratification is an abstract idea that's hard for some to grasp. When was the last time you were happy that something or someone, maybe you, was delayed?

"I'm stuck in traffic and will be delayed as a result, awesome!"

"There's a flight delay, and you're going to have to sleep in the airport, cool!"

"Your order was delayed at the warehouse, so the clothes won't arrive before your vacation, fabulous!"

Said no one, ever.

In the Spartan world, we have come to believe that in many cases, gratification is something that *must* be delayed to achieve success. This theory has been validated in the world of science, most notably in the form of what's famously called "the cookie experiment." Cookies? Baking goodies doesn't sound very Spartan, but it has everything to do with the Spartan mentality and the underpinnings of our philosophy. It's also one of the keys to unlocking success in life.

In 1972, a Stanford researcher by the name of Walter Mischel hatched an idea for an experiment that has since become famous and is studied and debated to this day. Mischel would give children their preferred treat: a marshmallow, a cookie, or a pretzel. He would tell them they could eat it right away — or wait fifteen minutes and eat two instead. A simple choice. He then tracked their subsequent success as the children matured into adulthood. As it turns out, those kids who refused the first cookie became more successful adults than those who took it. Cookie refusers became winners.

Jose Albanil, a graphic designer from Scottsdale, Arizona, knows what it's like to undergo the cookie test. He was training at Arizona Health and Fitness Expo, a Spartan-style workout facility, in anticipation of an upcoming race. After a warm-up, the trainer had him and the others do fifty squats, followed by thirty burpees, and then thirty planks-to-Supermans, a core and lower-back trial from hell. Then came sandbag carry-and-tosses around the building. "I was starting to sweat big time," says Jose. "My hands were so shaky I couldn't have held a cup of coffee if my life had depended on it at the moment."

His fellow trainees began to cut corners, missing reps and cutting short sets. In essence, those individuals were "taking the cookie." Jose was determined to complete the workout as it was being prescribed and reap the full benefits later. He did work smarter, though. He figured out that the farther he could throw his sandbag before picking it up, the faster he could go. It was harder to make those big tosses, and others chose not to. But he took the pain first for the reward later in true Spartan fashion. Who do you think's going to prevail out on the Spartan course, on a sports field, or in the boardroom — him or the people who took shortcuts and struggled along behind him regardless?

Carries over distance are one of my favorite obstacles for testing how someone would do on a cookie test. Your lungs are pumping hard, your legs are feeling like rubber, but you must keep going, carrying a large object whose weight is unevenly distributed. You're getting hit from all angles, and you can solve so many immediate discomforts and problems simply by dropping the object. But if you can just hold on, you can meet the challenge and reap the benefits of increased muscular endurance and grip strength.

I believe that the instant gratification that the cookie test measures is the number one reason we fail as humans in many aspects of our lives. To me there's no greater symbol of instant gratification in our society than the credit card. You don't actually have the money to purchase something, but you want it *now* anyway? No worries! Buy it now and repay it later; never mind that the interest payments may end up costing you twice the original amount. Our love affair with leverage was a major contributor to the financial crisis of 2008, and it's led to countless personal and family crises in households all over America.

I'm concerned with the havoc that repeatedly failing the cookie test can wreak on your life. All we have each day is *that day*, and we're not even guaranteed all twenty-four hours. The first cookie test you encounter each day comes when you wake up. If you decide to stay in bed for a while, you've already taken the cookie. But if you jump out of bed and embark upon a productive day, you postpone gratification until you've gained a head start. I'm convinced that the best way to start the day is with vigorous exercise. Grab a workout first thing, and it improves everything that follows. Do it every day, habitually, and you will change your life profoundly for the better.

How often do you take the cookie now? Do you wake up early in the morning and work out, or do you take the cookie and stay in bed? Do you take the cookie now and stay up all night drinking with friends, or go to bed early, wake up early, and take two cookies tomorrow by being more productive? If you finish the workout early and sleep enough, you'll enjoy many cookies later. The only way to teach the opposite is through experience — you need to feel just how bad it is when you don't stay on track and flunk a class or lose a valued customer. Conversely, you need to see how good it feels to nail it, to look in the mirror and see a six-pack, to have people tell you how great you look. In essence you're rewiring your brain.

Examples abound of people taking the cookie now with negative consequences, such as procrastinating in school or at work until a manageable task has turned into a crisis. You put off that term paper to party, but just think of the weight that would come off your shoulders if you had finished it early and turned it in. It's the same in the workplace. Think about what you need to accomplish each day, make a list, and get it done. Just because five o'clock is getting close doesn't mean you should give up and delay something until tomorrow. Push through until the end, check that item off your list, and start with a clean slate in the morning.

Even minor chores and tasks are well suited for the "take the cookie later" approach. Don't want to vacuum, clean the bathroom, or grocery shop? If tasks like these are left on the back burner, if you take the cookie now and relax, not only will the chores be harder when you eventually do them, but not having done them can complicate your day-to-day life. Rather buy a new pair of shoes than pay the electric bill on time? Put it off too long, and that bill will be way past due simply because you chose to forget about it for a week or two. You'll spend as much money on the late fee as you did on the shoes. Moments like these are perfect opportunities to embrace the "take the cookie later" mindset. Strive each day to finish what needs to get done, and your cookies will taste sweeter in the long run.

Science has found that the most successful people are not the most intelligent or the most talented but rather the ones who tough it out. Geoff Colvin, author of a book titled *Talent Is Overrated*, claims that the defining aspect of world-class performers isn't their talent but rather their devotion to regular practice. In *How Children Succeed*, Paul Tough compares GED recipients to high school graduates. In theory, they have equal intelligence and equivalent credentials, but high school graduates typically have higher incomes. Why? Because they had the drive to complete a task, in this case graduating from high school. Not that every kid who earned a GED punked out on high school — sometimes extenuating circumstances are to blame — but when they just quit, it appears to have a long-lasting effect.

In the same way, the kids who tough it out fifteen minutes to get the two cookies aren't necessarily extraordinarily intelligent. They just have what Angela L. Duckworth, PhD, a University of Pennsylvania researcher, calls grit. *Webster's Dictionary* defines *grit* as a "hard, sharp granule, an abrasive particle." Grit is used to smooth over a rough surface. A little grit in your sneaker can lead to bleeding blisters. In a person, it means unyielding and resolute. Grit is stick-to-it-iveness. You have to stick to it.

Spartans are gritty or they're not true Spartans. We accomplish our goals through persistent effort. Physical fitness and good health are not accomplished with a single, monumental effort. They are attained by consistent, focused, strenuous effort. I can think of more than a handful of individuals who had great talent in their sport and yet never attained the pinnacle of success in their career. Former NFL quarterback Jeff George, for example, had one of the best arms the league had ever seen. He practically had a rocket launcher attached to his right shoulder. Yet he bounced around from team to team and was never very successful at leading them to titles or even very many wins. He seemed to lack that intangible quality that Spartan-like quarterbacks such as Johnny Unitas, John Elway, and Tom Brady have had. He lacked their grit.

Then there are those with modest talent who nonetheless work on their skills and hone their talent through daily vigorous practice, over a long period of time, and become extremely successful as a result. Mariano Rivera, the retired New York Yankees closer, threw one pitch and only one pitch — a cut fastball — every game to the best hitters on earth. They knew it was coming every time. But he had perfected that one pitch through such dedicated practice that they still couldn't hit it. "Mo," as he was known, hung up his cleats as the best closer in the history of Major League Baseball. All based on the complete mastery of one pitch.

Grit isn't a short-term phenomenon. A conscientious, persistent athlete can achieve short-term goals such as improved fitness and weight loss. But grit is much more than that. Writing with three other researchers in a 2007 article published in the *Journal of Personality and Social Psychology*, Duckworth explained: "Grit entails working strenuously toward challenges, maintaining effort and interest over years despite failure, adversity, and plateaus in progress. The gritty individual approaches achievement as a marathon; his or her advantage is stamina."

If you're not gritty now, can grit rub off on you? Writing in a 2010 issue of the *Journal of Personality and Social Psychology*, a group of scientists at the University of California suggested that a person's personality tends to be stable over time. The cautious seventeen-year-old normally won't be wild and crazy in his or her fifties, the person who is risk averse won't evolve into a gambler, and so on. But it is important to understand that the environment can influence our behaviors. We may not be able to change our biology, but we do have the capacity to change our behaviors. We do have free will. In a similar vein, someone may have a genetic predisposition to develop heart disease, but if that person consciously chooses to eat healthfully, be physically active, and not smoke, heart disease is less likely to unfold.

For some, becoming gritty may be an easy transition. For others, it may require more conscious effort. Do you want more grit? Start here:

1. Write out your plan for success. Establish your baseline, set a goal, define a clear path toward that goal.
2. Share the plan. The recipient should be someone who is supportive yet can offer constructive criticism when needed. If necessary, hire a coach.
3. Eliminate distractions. What are your barriers? TV, Internet, video games?
4. Keep a journal of your successes and failures. Remember the

days when you would receive a gold star for exceptional performance in grade school? Give yourself a gold star for every success you have during the day.

5. Adjust as needed, as long as it doesn't diminish or change your original goal. Always work on solutions.

6. Last but not least, don't give up. Don't let setbacks become failures. Learn from them and keep moving forward. You must remain committed to your goals.

One of the reasons Spartan Races are so transformational is that participating in one takes you through the process of developing grit. It's like Grit 101. (1) You begin with the goal of completing a Spartan Race. (2) You tell your friends you're going to run it, maybe hire a trainer, or if not, find the information online. (3) You eliminate distractions by going to the gym instead of surfing Facebook; you stay on track with your diet by skipping Friday night happy hour with the coworkers. (4) You faithfully track your workouts, calories, and macronutrients. (5) Maybe you suffer an injury during your training. Instead of throwing in the towel, you make the necessary adjustments to keep pushing forward in a way that's safe and prudent. (6) You don't give up, even though occasionally you feel overwhelmed. Your stick-to-it-iveness extends to the race itself, especially the obstacle? These are the final tests of your will.

As you age, your ability to delay gratification can become second nature. You can go farther by actively attacking those things that you least want to do. To use a gym analogy, if you hate squats more than any other exercise, you will enter the gym and head straight to the squat rack, almost embracing the discomfort. If you go to work and have a to-do list twenty items deep, you tackle the most unappealing line item first — say, a call with a dissatisfied customer that you know will be difficult. Others will procrastinate, saving the most difficult for last. Unfortunately, the unpleasantness to come will weigh over them even while they are knocking out all the fun and easy tasks. When they finally get around to dealing with the tough task, it may well have gotten tougher, and there may well not be enough time to handle the situation. This ability to tackle difficulties head on can be learned and practiced. Don't despair that you're doomed to put things off because of a defective strand of DNA. It's just a bad habit that's formed over time, one that you can replace with much better habits.

From a distance, it becomes easy to see the benefits of delayed gratification. The problem is that most people fail to put it into practice when it becomes the real-world moment of decision. That's a major reason why I started organizing Spartan Races, to rip people out of their comfort zone, even if it meant thrusting them into chaos. The call of the race awakens something deep within.

Living Life on Your Own Terms

Every decision we make is based on delayed gratification and other Spartan concepts. Take this Spartan decision-making cheat sheet as an example. When the choice is:

1. Hard or soft on your children: almost always hard.
2. Work out or not when not feeling great: almost always yes.
3. Eat the dessert or not: always not.
4. Run a little farther when tired or not: almost always yes.
5. Step out of your comfort zone when you don't feel like it: always yes.

I learned a lot about time from an acquaintance of my father's named Big Phil. My father was a businessman, and it was very hard to do business in Queens if you weren't affiliated with certain people. Big Phil was one of those people. Big Phil had spent a lot of time in prison. He would take me to the store to buy groceries, and since the market was only a couple blocks away, he'd say, "Let's run!" I thought, Hey, why not? One day in a locker room, Big Phil started doing tai chi. That wasn't really something a guy did in Queens back then, but nobody said anything to him because he could have killed them. Big Phil taught me many things but chief among them: (1) Be extremely physical, and (2) use every minute of your time. My wife thinks I am nuts, but I will stretch or exercise in public places while I have time to kill. She gets embarrassed, for example, if I am doing burpees in an airport. But being healthy should never be embarrassing.

We are all creatures of habit to some degree. We all like some predictability. We know when to watch our favorite shows and when to arrive at the airport and when to brush our teeth. We go to work on Monday and sleep in on Saturday. Some go to church, some watch football. Life takes on a predictable cadence, and we slip into a comfort zone that feels like our everyday reality. We assume things will keep unfolding as we expect, that we'll eat another meal, live another day, and grab another paycheck, with nothing out of the ordinary derailing our steady progress. That is, until something derails it.

We often settle into these routines without really thinking about them, let alone analyzing their genesis. Then, one day, we wake up in a strange place, blink, and say, "How the hell did I get here? Have I been here this whole time?" It happens to the best of us. We become so comfortable that days blend into weeks, weeks into months, and, before we know it, we have sleepwalked through much our life. Many of us are sleeping now, and if we don't wake up soon, we may end up somewhere we didn't want to go, or worse, nowhere.

The "normal American life" is what we know and love. We *know* that we should drink soft drinks and eat pizza — that's what the people on TV and in magazines tell us we need. (They know best, after all.) We buy granola bars from the candy aisle. (Try again.) We buy ten different products for our hair because it's good for our scalp, and we sit and watch reality TV because that's what real life is like — never mind that it's more scripted than most dramas. We buy new phones and computers because, well, we have to stay up-to-date. We sit, we watch, and eventually we get cancer or some heart condition and die, an anonymous statistic. The cycle continues with our children, and their children, and their children. We think that's just the way things are.

Everyone says they don't have the time. Well, you have to make time. You need to add up all the hours in your day, as your day progresses, and see if you had thirty minutes where you could have done burpees, or walked, or done anything physical. I would be shocked if you could not find thirty minutes a day.

While sleepwalking through life, a person may unknowingly reject a golden opportunity. It might seem strange and unconventional, and therefore unsuited to "the way things really are." But could it be life is not as it should be? Could it be that life itself has gradually been covered and weighed down with something else, to the point where it is now completely hidden? Could it be that what we *thought* was life was keeping us from living this whole time? What could living be, anyway, if it's not this? So often the truth startles us, unsettles us, even terrifies us, because it clashes so violently with our neat and tidy opinions — our "normal" lives. It asks too much, we say. We'd have to change everything, so we shudder and retreat rather than steel our mind and advance. All because it's radically different, and therefore, it simply cannot be true.

As it turns out, so many things that we have conditioned ourselves to accept as fact may only indeed be hypothetical, if they are not completely false. The needs that "experts" claim we have may be less than needs, and the normal, pleasant life we thought we ought to live may in fact be the death of us. Our so-called needs for more things, more stuff, more space may in fact be constructions, ruses, and distractions from a deeper life where, no, *we don't need to buy all that.* The possessions stack much higher than our aim, when it should be the opposite. The fad diet books each praise a different vitamin and decry a different nutrient. "What is going on?" we ask ourselves. "Life could not possibly be *this* complicated."

When we are honest with ourselves, we know that something is off, but even so, we push it aside and try not to think about it. After all, how important could it be? It's not on the news. Our way of making habits causes us to believe, after a while, that change is quite impossible. Resigned to that thought, we wander on our way exactly as before, never changing, never changing, never changing. No movement, only stagnation.

I believe that life without change is death. The human body contains, on average, one hundred trillion cells, each of which is working frantically to outrun its impending disintegration. Every cell is constantly in motion: replenishing, rebuilding, maintaining, expanding. If they stopped for even one minute, we would vanish, a pile of lifeless chemicals. And so I've come to believe that life is movement, and movement is life. The thousands of people you see scrambling around the course on Spartan Race day, covered in mud, are alive and in the moment.

Deep inside each human being is a spirit that hungers for movement and for growth. A live and burgeoning ball of energy, the spirit naturally moves, expands, gyrates — dances, even — purely by virtue of its desire for freedom. It craves beauty over entertainment, meaning over triviality, and knowledge over sensation. American society devotes few harbors to the trade of truth. Too often we sacrifice the pursuit of knowledge, distracted instead by sparkling material things.

I believe we have a choice to make every day. We could choose to reject change, cling to our destructive habits, and continue ticking away the moments of our dull days in a steady march to death. It doesn't matter if we die tomorrow because nothing of note would happen in one day, ten days, or ten years.

Spartans choose to pivot their trajectory by choosing to do something that others view as outrageous and brave and different. "Life should not be a journey to the grave," said Hunter S. Thompson, "with the intention of arriving safely in a pretty and well preserved body, but rather to skid in broadside in a cloud of smoke, thoroughly used up, totally worn out, and loudly proclaiming, 'Wow! What a ride!'" Don't take this the wrong way. It doesn't mean to abuse yourself; it means to use up your time wisely—explore, create, and get what you want to get done in life done.

We all have a limited amount of time to spend on this planet, but if we spend it trying to live a normal life, I believe our time is wasted. To say something is normal is just a clever way of saying it makes no difference to anyone and changes nothing. Anyone can live this "normal" life, a life confined by someone else's boundaries. Anyone can live that way and, sadly, make no difference. We are all destined for the grave, but what a tragedy to arrive there without any scars, without any mark to show that we tried to do something amazing. Henry David Thoreau went to spend years in the woods because he didn't want to get to the end of his life and realize that he had "never lived." We, too, can take a step toward living and make our time count. We can start today.

Preparing for the unexpected is easy. You just need to do the unexpected. Break out of your routine. Go for a run at night. Swim in the open water. Stop and climb a hill in the distance. Go farther during that bike ride. When you stay within your own guardrails you are not preparing for the unexpected. So when you're finally confronted by it—and you will be—you won't know how to succeed.

4

CHANGING YOUR FRAME OF REFERENCE

The way to get started is to quit talking and begin doing.

— WALT DISNEY

THE FIRST SPARTAN Race was scheduled for May 2010 in Burlington, Vermont, near where we live, and I promoted it around the area through meetings that were held in local bars. A small group of college students grew really excited at the prospect and plastered posters all over the place encouraging people to join. Still, many people I spoke to didn't understand the basic concept.

"You mean like a triathlon?" someone asked.

"No, not really," I said. "More like a day in the military: You're either going to get kicked out or promoted."

Marketing was a challenge; after all, it was a brand-new product, and we were trying to convince people to come and get tortured, but that, no, really, it would be fun.

I remember saying to Andy, "I don't know if the world is ready for this."

Even though no one knew exactly what to expect, nearly seven hundred people signed up to compete in that first race, and with them came three hundred spectators, mostly friends and family members to cheer them on. On race day, most of the people who had entered, including the accomplished athletes, were somewhat skeptical. Every other race you sign up for defines the parameters: a marathon is a marathon, no matter what. A triathlon is running, biking, swimming every time. A hot dog eating contest is, well, a hot dog eating contest.

Yet that first Spartan Race was a completely new experience for every participant, and for us, it was a wild experiment conducted in the lab of the wilderness and fueled by the human spirit. That race, and the ones that followed in those early days, were part adventure race, part Spartan battle, and full-on spectacle. The first field of entrants was a motley crew, a mix of athletes and friends. It looked like a scene from that Mel Gibson movie *Braveheart*, with people of all shapes and sizes dressed up in crazy-looking attire.

At the starting line of that first race, folks were nervous. Many had never done anything like this before and clearly had no idea what they had gotten themselves into. We didn't know for certain if people were actually going to move forward when the starting gun went off.

Almost immediately, competitors were dropped into waist-deep ice-cold water. Within twenty minutes, anger was visible on the faces of some competitors' faces. But almost all of them stuck it out, kept going, and it was only at the finish line that the smiles burst out. It was like children had taken over adult bodies. I remember thinking, Is Vermont unique or is something going on here?

Trepidation, suffering, anger, then love! That's how the average person still encounters and becomes acclimated to the Spartan Race.

After that, the Spartan Race took hold really quickly and growth came fast, and "why" is a good question. A lot of it has to do with the personal, almost spiritual connection brought about through the Spartan Races. My childhood was in many ways troubled, but I've taken my father and mother's best values and combined them to make a nearly metaphysical connection to Spartan participants, while also exposing them to the results of work that transcends what any of them thought possible. This is what sets them on fire, makes them become über-fans, and prompts them to post across social media, turning Spartan Race into a phenomenon. I was just lucky and savvy enough to recognize this response and validate and celebrate the loyalty of my followers.

This loyalty has made the business proliferate, growing to more than one hundred races in only four years. My partners and I have staged races in front of tens of thousands of people in faraway places like Slovakia and in cool stadiums, including Citi Field and Fenway Park, in the shadow of the Green Monster. Three hundred thousand people a day follow daily workouts that we post on spartan.com and blast out across our social media platforms. After mixed martial arts, obstacle racing is the world's fastest-growing sport. Only people don't watch these races; they participate in them.

At every step along the way, we've changed our own frame of reference as a business as our customers have changed theirs. It's been a Herculean task, day after day, to build this organization to the point where putting on one hundred events in seventeen countries in one season is even possible. For a while, I was receiving four-hundred-plus e-mails a day. I felt like I was living in a pinball machine, and I was the ball. Finally, though, things started to flow and take shape and processes began to take hold.

I don't want to say we've become mainstream because, in many ways, we are a reaction against the mainstream. But we are in no way fringe, either. Spartan Race is now a big, popular business, and we're just getting started. We are changing lives daily. Participants e-mail us, Tweet, and Facebook us about how transformative an experience it was for them. One guy showed up at the farm unannounced, and Courtney freaked out because she thought he was there to rob us. As a matter of fact, he just wanted to thank me for changing his life.

Our grip could have loosened at any moment, but we held on

and kept going. Our best marketing was word-of-mouth based. Our converts spread the word for us. By the end of 2013, Spartan Races attracted more than 650,000 entrants, including elite, professional, and amateur athletes, and the sport of obstacle racing was finding a growing and devoted community.

In August 2013, we held our thirty-fifth race of the season forty minutes outside of Salt Lake City at a scenic venue called Soldier Hollow. The course was nestled up against a mountain, and from a distance, you could see streams of racers moving in small groups up and down the trails, like ants scrambling around a picnic.

This particular race was a Spartan Beast. As the name suggests, it's one of our toughest events, with thirteen-plus miles of trail snaking up and down a mountainside, punctuated by twenty-five obstacles along the way. Each obstacle included an athletic element, a requirement for all of our courses. We don't shock people with electric wires or place obstacles designed purely for a cheap thrill. We run competitions, not an amusement park. Over the course of this race, participants would be throwing a spear at a target thirty feet away, like humans did to hunt; rolling under barbed wire; sloshing around in mud pits; and carrying large objects over distances.

That's just the tip of the iceberg. Depending on their conditioning level, the racers would spend three to five hours busting their ass in the boiling sun. Sound crazy? Andy and I would often say when training: "The ancient Spartans had it a lot tougher than this!"

For the elite Spartan athletes, this is a serious race, and they're not messing around. But you'll also see less serious athletes, people for whom this is a moment of personal triumph. Maybe it's the culmination of a weight-loss transformation, or something a father and his teenage daughter decided to do together before she heads off to college. A lot of racers are laughing and smiling, clearly enjoying themselves despite all the hard work and the obstacles. At one of the mud pits at Soldier Hollow, a girl in her teens crawls through mud and up onto a berm, where she looks over at what appears to be her mother holding a camera. The girl smiles, throws a sign, and hits a quick bodybuilder pose while her mom clicks away. Then she hops down into the mud on the other side and continues with the race.

Over at another mud pit, racers climb ropes in an attempt to ring a bell, signifying success. The three people doing sloppy-looking burpees off to the side reveal that not everyone reaches the top. Even for those who do, this is a genuine struggle. We're used to seeing professional athletes on TV and at events, and even when they lose, there's a certain grace and fluidity about what they're doing — after all, they're athletes. But here, you often see average people grunting and sweating their way through occasionally awkward situations. They trip, stumble, and fall, only to get back up and trudge forward. Kind of how life often unfolds.

There are genuine risks and real injuries that happen, too. At one obstacle, people are carrying heavy objects back and forth when a guy turns his ankle, causing him to buckle and crash to the ground, where he writhes as his friends call for help. There's a medical team at every race, and they're summoned to help this competitor, who is clearly injured and in pain.

After the fallen receives medical attention, I chat with a guy named Aziz Alhazeem, who, it turns out, has flown fifteen hours from Kuwait, where he serves in that country's national guard. "I cannot find that kind of race in my country, so I have to travel," he says, when asked why he was willing to travel so far for what some folks would liken to torture. Having completed the race, Aziz was heading back to Kuwait the next morning, mission accomplished. That guy is a true Spartan.

Staring Down Death Like a Spartan

Every race and its obstacles reshapes each race participant's life. Sometimes, these changes are profound. Spartan competitor Jim Mullane is also a cancer survivor. In September 2001, Mullane was diagnosed with non-Hodgkin lymphoma, which is cancer of the white blood cells. His cancer was stage four, meaning that it was advanced. His doctors had told him he probably had only six to eight years left to live. A year of intensive chemotherapy relegated his cancer to full remission. Unfortunately, it returned soon after that. "I had four additional types of treatments spread over four years, until I finally reached a sustainable remission and enjoyed living cancer-free for five years," Mullane explained. He took advantage of this reprieve, fathering two daughters with his wife, Lori.

Mullane relapsed in early 2011, ten years later, and had to resume treatment. He also decided to make major lifestyle changes to bolster his immune system; after all, he now had two young lives depending on his own. He cleaned up his diet until most of his calories were coming from fruits, vegetables, and lean proteins. He gave up alcohol and sugary drinks in favor of water and green tea.

Then he made an even bolder life decision: he would attempt a three-mile Spartan Race, which required him to push his body. The militaristic trappings of the Spartan idea appealed to him, given that he was in a fight to save his life. He signed up for the Pennsylvania Spartan Sprint and hooked up with a group of Spartan Elite members for his training. Every Wednesday morning, they'd meet up and run the mountains of Valley Forge, Pennsylvania. According to the scans he'd periodically receive, his disease was holding stable.

Until it wasn't. Recalls Mullane: "The Thursday before the race, I had a routine treatment and checkup, and the doctors found 'notable' growths in the lymph nodes in both my neck and groin. They scheduled me for an emergency PET scan on Friday afternoon, so my pre-race fuel-up was an eighteen-hour fast! Thankfully, the scan results, while showing cancer progression, also showed slow growth involvement."

Mullane lined up for the 10:45 heat that Saturday morning having slept only two hours the night before. Participants would agree afterward that the course's relentless inclines would make this the hardest sprint to date. Nonetheless, Mullane powered through to the finish line, finishing thirty-ninth in his age group with a time of one hour and twenty-four minutes.

We say that you'll know at the finish line, and Mullane did. "The feeling when crossing that finish line was amazing," he says. "It felt great to conquer the mountain and share the experience with some amazingly motivated people. There are parallels between my cancer battle and a Spartan Race. They are mentally and physically challenging and, when you want to succeed, both require an enormous amount of courage and strength and perseverance."

This is a great example of a man changing his frame of reference in the face of an enormous obstacle. His battle against this disease continues — Mullane began a five-month cycle of chemotherapy in August 2013 — but he continues to stare down this foe with optimism and determination. "I will not and cannot quit fighting."

There are less-dramatic settings in which you can change how you view both your circumstances and the world around you. Andy has a cousin who was born a week after me. Let's call him John. As I'm writing this passage, John and I are both forty-three years old, but we have traveled very different paths in life. He works on Wall Street and makes a shitload of money. John's weight grew as fast as his wealth, though, and he ballooned up to 280 pounds. He made some money, but he did so at the expense of his health and quality of life. He had a driver take him to his office on Wall Street even though he only lived a mile and a half away. He could have walked to work every day, and his life would have changed if only he had done so. When he needed a break, he went outside and smoked a cigarette. He and his wife enjoyed fine dining with no regard for the extravagant calories. He almost never exercised.

John always seemed pissed off about something. He told me, "You have no idea how stressful my job is." His five brothers, who are all fit, always said to me, "Why don't you talk to him? He won't listen to us." I didn't want to hurt his feelings and say what I thought, which was, "You're fat, and you need to take care of yourself." So finally, I nicely suggested that he join the gym and get a trainer. He said, "You have no idea how embarrassing it is at 280 pounds to walk into a gym. You've got this maniac doing burpees, you got the girl in the sports bra with the ripped stomach, you got the muscle head over there benching. What am I going to do? It's embarrassing."

Eventually, though, I convinced John to change his ways. First he got on the treadmill at home and started walking, and then he started lifting. He cut back on his smoking, and in a matter of months, he had lost nearly forty pounds.

Amazing what you can do if you want to change your life. If you *don't*, your life is just going to stay the same until it eventually gets worse. John recently told me, "Man, I feel so good. I always walk home from work, and I don't smoke as much as I used to." His stress release has gone from a smoke to a walk; that one simple change has set in motion a process that vaporized almost forty pounds. This is not a full-blown Spartan mindset, but it's the inklings of what puts you on the path.

John's experience illuminates a valuable lesson. Human beings, like all animals, are creatures of habit. Not only do we develop behaviors of action, we also develop patterns of expectation. Based on prior experience, we establish our frame of reference, and we look at everything through that prism. But that doesn't mean it's reality. We simply have elevated it to that status.

Compare the satisfaction of eating a banana after Thanksgiving dinner to eating a banana after a weeklong fast. When not eating, we gradually grow accustomed to being hungry; we recalibrate our frame of reference. After not eating for a week, you would think anything that's edible tastes like a gourmet meal. The reverse holds true. Look at the guy who eats in world-class restaurants every night. Let's say his hundred-dollar steak is cooked medium instead of medium rare, or one of the brussels sprouts was slightly undercooked. Well, the chef ruined his evening. This guy has become used to such luxurious cuisine that he can't tolerate anything less.

Money does not equal happiness, and too many people strive for wealth as a way to achieve happiness. A Spanish economist named Manel Baucells Alibes wanted to answer this question: why are millionaires living in mansions in the United States not infinitely happier than Masai warriors living in huts in Kenya? Alibes developed a mathematical formula:

Happiness = What I Have Now – What I Had Before

Creatures of habit get used to everything, including the greatest pleasures. What was once a luxury becomes a convenience, and what was once a convenience becomes a need. Eventually, everything in our lives starts to "suck," because we are continuously bored or dissatisfied with what we have.

Society teaches us to respond to this dissatisfaction by accumulating more. We will be happy if only we get a raise, if only we get the latest gadget, if we get a bigger house. Let's say that, by some stroke of fate, we do get our raise, our new toy, or our new house, then for a while, we love life. What we have now is greater than what we had before. So we are happy.

Fast forward. We have grown accustomed to our new salary, to our new toys, to our new house. What we have now is equal to what we had before, so we are no longer happy. The quest for more and more stuff, for more and more pleasure — all it does, ultimately, is raise our expectations for more and more material stimulation. It becomes harder and harder, and more expensive, to stay content. Did you ever wonder why lots of billionaires seem unhappy, if not miserable? Spartans don't fall into this trap; we take the opposite approach. If "Happiness" equals "What I Have Now" minus "What I Had Before," how can we use this to our advantage? We do this by controlling our frame of reference.

Reset Your Frame of Reference

I use daily intense exercise as one way to reset my frame of reference. My mom would reset hers every day by meditating. People may have thought, She's just sitting there doing nothing. Yet the science has caught up and discovered that meditation can make people happier by increasing their pain threshold and releasing feel-good chemicals in the brain. By sitting in quiet stillness for an hour every morning, people can recalibrate their brains. The internal chatter they've grown accustomed to hearing in their minds seems noisy in comparison to their meditation time. So they reorganize their thought patterns to keep the mind quieter throughout the day.

The development of mental control is the foundation for building an unbeatable mind that will not fail at any worthy goal or task, including a Spartan Race. I'm not talking about developing psychic powers like bending spoons. I'm talking about learning to block out distractions so you can focus enough to operate at an elite level, whatever your goals may be. Your monkey mind refers primarily to your rational, analytical "left brain" mind, especially if it is untrained through higher education and deep concentration. It is estimated that this part of our brain accounts for roughly 12 percent of our total thinking power. The other 88 percent lies in our creative subconscious, our "right brain," and is poorly engaged by the majority of people.

The first step for developing mental control is silencing yourself enough so you can witness what is going on in your head. As you witness, you gain awareness of the external and internal influences that cause the chatter. The silence is the first layer of training for the mind. Gaining the space to witness our thoughts tames them in the process. We begin to bring our mind back under our control, allowing ourselves longer periods of focus. Then, we have the possibility of removing negative distractions and ensuring that our psychology supports our physiology. Sometimes it's as simple as breathing deeply, holding for a period, and then releasing slowly.

Epictetus, the great Stoic, defined wealth not as having numerous and extravagant possessions, but as having few wants. When you've been to hell and back, food, water, and shelter will suffice to make you happy. It was only after I was broke that I started to appreciate every dollar I had. Working hard all week makes us thankful for Friday. Winter makes us appreciate spring. We need an appropriate frame of reference in order to be happy. The key to true happiness, therefore, is regularly recalibrating your frame of reference. It makes life simpler, healthier, and more enjoyable.

If you think you can't compete in a Spartan race then you should meet Spartan Racer Misty Diaz, who was born with spina bifida, a congenital birth defect in which vertebrae in the spinal cord don't fuse properly. "I remember driving around in Long Beach and finally seeing a sign for the Ronald McDonald 5K walk," she recalled. "They'd helped my family in the past, so I thought: What better way to give back? So I signed up, and doing it felt wonderful. Which made me think: If I can walk a 5K, I can run one. A week later, I signed up for the Seal Beach 5K run, despite the fact that I can only walk using canes. I used Google to find training regimens and started hitting the gym regularly. I completed that race, and I've now completed thirty-two endurance races. My current goal—which I've almost accomplished—is running three half marathons. I signed up for three that are scheduled within a month."

Next up is a Spartan Sprint in Malibu, California. "You'd think I would have had enough discomfort after twenty-eight operations for spina bifida," she says, laughing. "But I love training, and I want to test my limits, so what better challenge than trying a Spartan Race? The hardest part for all of us is convincing our minds what our bodies are capable of. Many train the body but forget to train the mind. I know I can do a Spartan Race. I'm just going to have to turn on a different type of 'beast mode!'"

This is the stuff that continues to motivate me. I believe such greatness lies within all of us, albeit too often hidden. The stories of Mullane and Diaz are amazing in that each individual overcame an immense physical obstacle to take control of their body and run or, in Diaz's case, plan for a Spartan Race. When extreme events become your "new normal," you develop something greater than endurance, and you learn about more than mere survival. You develop a new ability to make clear judgments even during unclear circumstances.

I started Spartan Race as a way to find amazing people. What I didn't realize was that finding amazing people would be a thrilling dividend to starting Spartan Race, one that continues to energize and remotivate me, just as it is doing the same for so many participants.

Spartan Up! Life Lesson No. 2: Everyone Matters

During my second month of college, our professor gave us a pop quiz. I had studied hard and breezed through the questions until I read the last one: "What is the first name of the woman who cleans the school?"

Surely this was some kind of joke. I had seen the cleaning woman several times. She was tall, dark haired, and in her fifties, but how would I know her name? So I handed in my paper with the last question blank. As we were being dismissed, one student asked if the last question would count toward our quiz grade. "Absolutely," said the professor. "In your careers, you will meet many people. All are significant. They deserve your attention and care, even if all you do is smile and say 'Hello.'"

I've never forgotten that lesson. Her name was Susan.

5

GETTING SPARTAN FIT

> I hated every minute of training, but I said, "Don't quit. Suffer now and live the rest of your life as a champion."
>
> — MUHAMMAD ALI

IF YOU SAW the movie *300*, you may remember the early scenes involving a child being cast out into the wilderness to fend for himself. The barren landscape was forbidding, and if the boy wanted to survive, he'd have to use his ingenuity and courage. At one point, he comes face to face with a savage-looking beast. I won't give away the scene, but the kid does his best to rise to the occasion without an Xbox or a McDonald's Quarter Pounder. Somehow he survives.

In ancient times, Spartan males were all considered eligible soldiers who might be called upon to defend the city-state. This doctrine required early physical and mental preparation, and soldiering became a man's profession. Their existence centered on defending the Spartan way of life—for their entire life.

How would our children, some of them raised on video games and junk food, stack up going hand-to-hand against these young Spartans in the wilderness? Our kids don't wrestle with beasts; they waddle through elementary school overweight and lazy, opting for the extra cupcake rather than the extra mile. Twenty-three percent of America's adolescents have either pre-diabetes or type 2 diabetes. Meanwhile, 69 percent of adults in the US are overweight or obese. Associated with this state are life-threatening ailments such as heart disease, stroke, type 2 diabetes, and certain types of cancer. This has become the new normal for us as a society. No wonder our kids are falling into that same health trap.

Entitlement and overindulgence come out of the epidemic of divorce in the past few decades, and the intensification of fear of the outdoors has proliferated through the pervasive bad news on twenty-four-hour cable networks. This has led to parents "making up" for misfortune and absenteeism with hyperindulgence and hyper-reward. Or conversely, with an overpresence and hyperprotectiveness embodied in the term "helicopter parents"—those who refuse to let their kids outside of the house by themselves. Levels of anxiety about nature and the outdoors have risen measurably in young people. So they're apt to stop asking to go out there and stay in their rooms.

These are the exact issues we have successfully addressed with Spartan Race. We're giving people what they need because the world has dropped out of balance for so many of them.

To move freely, to breathe fully and deeply, and to have the ability to surmount physical obstacles is a privilege. A Spartan knows this to the core of his or her being, and, as a result, makes his or her physical health a top priority. You can talk all you want about mental strength and a positive attitude, but the Spartan ideal as we embody it comes from physical fitness. Mind over matter only takes you so far before you find yourself beyond your body's literal physical capacity. A disembodied brain cannot scale an eight-foot wall. You can't light up a smoke or develop a beer belly and call yourself a Spartan. You can't sit for five years watching television and eating Cheetos and then suddenly go out and do an ultramarathon or a Spartan Race, or anything nearly as demanding. You're kidding yourself if you think otherwise. You have to put in the effort.

All of the sitting of modern life is an outright denial of true nature. We are animals, after all. We are evolved to run and jump and climb, throw spears, fight, and dance. Our bodies were built to move — that's why we have brains in the first place — yet somehow we ended up sitting for hours on end. Exercise is the best defense you have against anxiety, stress, depression, and a whole host of other diseases. It helps cells repair themselves, and it quite literally heals the effects of stress through the release of something called brain-derived neurotrophic factor, or BDNF. Researchers have found, not surprisingly, that when students exercise regularly, their stress levels drop. Upset? Stressed? Mad? Run. Still feel that way? Run faster. You've got nothing to lose but weight and stress. Regular exercise is just as effective as drugs for controlling panic disorders. No wonder employees who exercise call in sick fewer days than employees who don't.

It's been said that there is no telling how many miles you will have to run while chasing a dream. But running great distances or crushing the weights for an hour straight takes more than desire and intestinal fortitude. It takes a strong heart, trained lungs, and powerful metabolic machinery, such as mitochondria and oxidative enzymes, working at full force. Developing that internal horsepower requires consistent training. As a result, people who are obese and sedentary don't respond to a single bout of exercise nearly as robustly as people who are already trained. It's ironic, but when it comes to exercise, the rich grow richer. No wonder so many people who are out of shape stay that way. It can be harder for them than it is for the already fit. They may start with good intentions, but slow initial progress can result in a negative feedback loop. Unfortunately, the couch potato has become America's majority. There are more fat people than there are Republicans, Democrats, Independents, Christians, Jews, Muslims, Buddhists, or any other group. And their ranks, like their waistlines, swell by the day.

The vast majority of chronic disease in America is preventable if we avoid a sedentary lifestyle, stop smoking cigarettes, and start eating better. But it's remarkable how slow we as a society have been in recognizing this epidemic and doing something about it. That's tragic because your own fitness is one thing you have full control over, and your fitness level holds tremendous sway over your long-term health.

If you think back to your childhood, you worked out all day. Only you didn't think of it as working out. Whether you called it play, or recess, or hanging out with your friends, you were running around outside, climbing trees, swinging from branches, tossing snowballs, crawling around in the mud, and doing all sorts of other things you weren't supposed to do. The harder, the messier, the more competitive the activity, the more you enjoyed doing it. When dusk settled, you finally had to go in for dinner because if you didn't, your mom would remind you who the boss was. But you didn't want it to end. You wanted to keep playing, to keep exercising, until you couldn't play or exercise any longer. Finally, when you arrived home, exhaustion and hunger would hit. Only then would you fall asleep. You wouldn't need a pill or scented candles to help you do it; your body worked the way it was meant to work.

We learned things about the world around us and ourselves by testing our limits. You mother might have told you for years that it was dangerous to swim right after eating, until that day when you decided to rebel and swim thirty minutes after lunch. You didn't die, randomly burst into flames, or suffer any other ill consequences.

Remember how amped you felt as a kid when you saw a set of monkey bars on the playground? That was a challenge. Even the name conjured the sort of mischievous fun that held sway over a young mind. If someone had taken the trouble to erect the apparatus, hell, you were going to use it. Cleaning your room or doing yard work was a chore; the monkey bars, those were fun. If your grip gave way halfway across and you fell down in a sandpit below, so what? That was fun, too. If your hands developed calluses, no problem. They were badges of honor.

I would argue that treating our kids as if they need to be covered in Bubble Wrap throughout childhood has a downside. They grow up divorced from the natural world around them and fearful of anything even mildly threatening. Without question, kids who are allowed to play freely may scrape a knee, lose a tooth, and maybe even break a bone in unfortunate circumstances. Part of growing up is taking some risks and learning their consequences, good and bad. If you take someone who wasn't allowed to play outside as a child and place them in an obstacle race, they'll be ill prepared to deal with any of the obstacles that appear before them.

The monkey bars present an awesome physical challenge for children and adults alike. They tax your grip strength, challenge your arms, leave your back muscles screaming for mercy, test your core's ability to keep you stable. You may feel like you're back on the playground in elementary school, but for many racers, this is one of the toughest obstacles they face. You have to dig deep and hold on tight and test your overall muscular endurance. To quote the late football player and professional wrestler Alex Karras, "Toughness is in the soul and spirit, not in muscles."

The race is only the culmination of our physical training. It is a place to test how you are living your life. The Greek philosopher Aristotle knew that mastering self-discipline unlocked success. The Spartan plan wrings every ounce of what life has to offer, and it's based on principles that have been known only to the enlightened since ancient times. With our accelerating desire for everything faster, easier, cheaper, we've lost sight of these ancient tenets. To rediscover and embrace them is to give our mind, body, and spirit the chance to flourish as one. At that point, anything becomes possible.

Survival of the Fittest

The Spartan idea of fitness may not resemble yours. We do things differently. We're more likely to be training outside than inside, more likely to be using our own body than weights for resistance, less likely to be resting during our workouts.

Military organizations often train this way out of necessity — when you're deployed, you may not have access to a gym in the conventional sense. But Jack LaLanne pioneered this no-frills style of fitness a half century ago, delivering workouts into living rooms across America for free. I was recently visiting with Jack LaLanne's wife. "La La," he called her. She's eighty-eight years old, and she dropped down and gave me ten pushups. She was not performing magic; she was performing like a human should — a human who ate healthy foods and exercised her whole life.

Gadgets aren't the only shortcut today. We all know that body-building drugs are a shortcut to size. Steroids, growth hormone, and various illegal substances can help make you much more muscular. But at what cost to your health? Years off your life, many would argue. There is no shortcut: if you exercise often and eat healthfully, lasting long-term results will follow.

The endurance world hasn't been immune to such cheating. In fact, cycling at the Tour de France level is arguably the only sport whose use of performance-enhancing drugs (PEDs) is as widespread as that of professional bodybuilding. By now everyone knows about Lance Armstrong's comeuppance, and all the deception and intimidation he mustered to protect his secretive use of PEDs over many years. Such duplicity and the dishonor it produces is the antithesis of the Spartan creed. Our lifestyle pits you against your past self and your former limitations, so drug-taking would defeat the purpose of what we do.

We believe that all you need to become fit is intestinal fortitude and the willingness to train. Equipment or drugs should not make the difference. The whole point of Spartan racing is to summon something deep within you in the heat of battle and competition. We take your comfort zone and surround it with yellow tape, like cops would do at a crime scene to keep people out.

We train to compete in our own races. This provides a sense of purpose, a community for accountability's sake, and benchmarking to know how you're stacking up not only against others but against yourself. The simple act of signing up for a race is a powerful incentive. We encourage folks to pick an event with a hard deadline and stick to it. A race isn't the only goal you could set, though. It could be weight loss or finding exercise you love to do.

The key to staying motivated is the prospect of either a reward or a consequence. We encourage you to tell all your friends so they'll help you stay in shape. And you'll be motivated by the sheer fact of not wanting to fail at something you have told them you are trying. Over time, this level of commitment, the signing up *and* following through, extends to other aspects of your life. Eventually you'll find yourself saying things like, "I have made a commitment to myself. The rest of my life I'm going to stay fit." You're no longer willing to negotiate with yourself. You've decided to run up the hill so one doesn't appear on your midsection.

Healthy athletic competition as a means of learning seems more and more alien where it's most needed, that is, in our school systems. Andy Weinberg, whom I introduced earlier, spent considerable time teaching at a small liberal arts school. He often received e-mails from parents expressing complaints such as, "I have a question about this grade. My son said he did great and for some reason only got a C in this class, when he should've gotten a B. Can you give me a call and talk about this?"

Andy's standard response? "Your child is twenty years old. He or she is an adult. They're in college. Let them plead their own case if they disagree."

I'll give you an example of what I'm talking about. There was a football player at the same college with a nose for trouble, including partying in the dorms past curfew, for which he was busted. His grades were subpar, too. He was your classic screw off. So his mom sent this long e-mail to the college president, the dean of students, the coach, *and* the kid's academic advisor, the gist of it being: "You should be ashamed of yourself. When my son came to college, you were supposed to look after him. This is an embarrassment to my husband and me that he earned Cs in his classes."

The dean didn't even bother responding, the letter was so ridiculous. The coach replied: "I'm sick to my stomach that I'm even reading this e-mail. At some point in life, your son needs to take responsibility for his actions. You need to cut the apron strings. He's twenty years old, for crying out loud!"

Even when the kids at this college would take the initiative, the conversations often betrayed a deep sense of entitlement. Other professors would tell Andy that kids would come to them and say: "If you have a moment, Professor, I'd like to discuss my grade. How did I earn a B? I've never had a B in my life."

My friend would reply: "A is for excellent. You're a good student. You're a smart guy. But you're not excellent, at least not yet, anyway."

Hearing an honest answer like that would crush many of these kids. They'd probably been patted on the back and stroked their whole life, regardless of what they had achieved. "To try" becomes synonymous with "to succeed." I bet you they had always been told they were excellent. However, at a college with strong academics, they were good, but they weren't excellent, something the professor would explain: "It's different here. Here's what I'm looking for. If you want to turn in a ten-page paper and receive an A, it needs to be unbelievable. Yours wasn't."

Today we shower kids with plaques, certificates, and even trophies for nothing: "Congrats, kid, you showed up! You're so great!" Never mind that the kid didn't do shit. Just so he or she got equal playing time. Even at the high school level, kids are often put in the game only because they need their turn to play. I'm okay with that for junior high school, recreational leagues, summer camps, and similar settings, but when you're playing at the varsity level in high school, play to win or lose. Yes, it's a team sport, but the goal of the team is to win, not to let everybody play. Your son or daughter may not be good enough. That's okay. I'm not saying he or she isn't a great person, but maybe they haven't yet put in the amount of work that they need to in order to succeed. Yet no one wants to hear that anymore. It's hard for parents to swallow the reality that their child simply *isn't* the best.

Imagine if we ran the Death Race this way. What if everybody got a skull that day, no matter what? What would be the motivation then? If everyone gets a trophy regardless, why should anyone try hard? The same goes at Spartan Race. We don't reward people for trying. We run the only obstacle race where you get a penalty for failing an obstacle. You don't get a prize before you finish. If you quit, you don't get a medal. You didn't earn it.

I don't want to be rewarded with a trophy when I don't achieve my goal. I don't want to be protected from that pain. If I get a trophy when I fail, then I'm going to believe that I performed at the peak of my ability. And that may prevent me from getting better. This is basic psychology. Rewarding behavior only regenerates the behavior. Rewarding habitual failure breeds a character of failure. What kind of attitude are we encouraging when we give everyone a trophy? We're encouraging an attitude of self-congratulation that leads to apathy, where accomplishments are meaningless and hard work is beside the point. The pain of regret, the pain of failure — the drive to avoid feeling this pain ever again is what pushes us to work harder, to be a better person. No failure is so great that we cannot learn from it. No mistake is so pitiful that we have to spend the rest of our lives wallowing in the mud. Spartans are resilient! We fight to recover what we have lost, and we do so relentlessly.

Unlike today's parenting model of coddle and comfort, the Spartans thrust adversity upon their kids. In ancient times, the concept of learning how to "fail well" encouraged young Spartans to develop critical skills of resiliency and self-determination. For example, Spartan boys were traditionally provided less food than necessary, forcing them to acquire what they needed. I often train on little to no food myself, other than drinking some coconut water during an extended workout. Just like the Spartans, I'm training my body to work through pain and discomfort. Only by placing ourselves in a state of disequilibrium can we grow stronger and tougher.

So you know that we like to compete, but what else defines the Spartan approach to fitness? Let me outline several key points:

Spartans like to train outdoors. Outside the confines of the gym the landscape is (gasp!) unpredictable. Rocks, leaves, hills, trees, grass, mud — all these elements translate into uneven and challenging terrain, and ultimately pay off big in terms of workout benefits: continual balance adjustments in the ankles and knees work the smaller, supporting muscles and ligaments of your lower body as well as engaging the core. Uneven terrain also makes your brain work harder, requiring you to focus on each step you take to make adjustments in your stride and pace according to the surface. You expend more energy (read: calories) running or hiking outside than you do when striding along on a flat treadmill because of all these additional muscular requirements. You don't get better at running hills by walking on the treadmill.

Science has identified other advantages to exercising outdoors. Being outside can give your mood a supercharge, according to one study from the Peninsula College of Medicine and Dentistry. Researchers discovered that those who exercised outdoors experienced an improvement in well-being and a reduction in the symptoms of depression. Subjects also felt revitalized, had a decrease in tension, and experienced elevated self-esteem, as compared with those who exercised indoors. Aside from its bronzing capabilities, sunlight is a natural mood enhancer, boosting serotonin levels, enhancing feelings of calmness and heightening your senses.

Fresh-air training is also green, meaning no electricity used, no water wasted, and the footprints you leave behind are human footprints, not carbon. Finally, training outside requires no gym dues, no towel service, no expensive smoothies or overpriced water — just you, your shoes, and the great outdoors.

Spartans often train together, but they don't need to. Many of my greatest endurance feats have been accomplished in isolation. At the same time, I also do many endurance events with a partner or as part of a team. In the morning I usually work out with Andy, who lives next door and will knock on my door at 4:00 AM. We're both incredibly driven and disciplined, and we feed each other's drive during these workouts. You may have experienced the same sort of mutually beneficial relationship with a training partner at your gym or with someone who would run with you in preparation for a 10K or a marathon.

A good training partner can push you farther and faster when things are going well, but they can become essential when you're burned out on training or skipping workouts and starting to slack.

You are conspiring against your own laziness by having a friend help hold you accountable to your fitness goals.

Spartans don't train in ways that are too specific and specialized. We've all seen the cyclist with skinny arms who looks like a quad monster from the waist down. We've seen the bodybuilder with perfectly proportioned musculature who couldn't run around the block if he or she had to. Neither of those individuals would fare well in a Spartan Race.

For decades the fitness movement revolved around going to the gym to train certain body parts on certain days: chest day, leg day, and so forth. This is how professional bodybuilders train to this day. Onstage, after all, they're judged on the size and aesthetics of each body part in relation to the other. These athletes would present their body part workouts in issues of *Muscle & Fitness* and other magazines, and fitness hopefuls would dutifully trudge off to the gym to emulate them.

Unfortunately, this sort of training doesn't have much carryover to the real world. There is no life situation that requires you to do multiple reps of leg extensions, unless you're doing leg extensions at the gym. In no way does it prepare you for the unexpected situations that life presents: a kid in one arm, a grocery bag that's spilling over in the other arm, and a patch of mud that sends you lurching in one direction, requiring every muscle in your body to clench at once.

A Spartan Race is designed to incorporate as many of these challenges as possible. Once a racer is tired, muddy, and dispirited, even we can't predict how he or she will respond to the unexpected alchemy of these diverse elements.

Spartans need muscular endurance more than they need huge muscles. Powerlifters, other strength athletes, and even some bodybuilders focus on what's called a one-rep max: the amount of weight they lift for one and only one repetition. They would fail on a second rep were they to attempt it. I struggle to see how useful this is in the real world and everyday life. Maybe when someone's pulling a car off of another person, or some other crazy one-time situation? We very rarely need one-rep max strength for anything.

In the Spartan world, we focus on developing strength that can be sustained over time and many repetitions. We climb ropes dangling above mud pits. We carry heavy, uneven loads across rutted, rocky fields. We scale walls and then propel ourselves to the other side. Sometimes we carry or help each other, much like soldiers assist each other on the battlefield. You can see it in the physiques on the Spartan courses on race day. Not that heavily muscled men and women don't do our races, but for the most part, our elite racers are lean athletes. These people look fit and great, but for the most part, these are "go" muscles, not "show" muscles.

Spartan fitness is different from bodybuilding. It bears more resemblance to something like CrossFit, with its emphasis on functional training and full-body movements, as well as its disdain for machines. Indeed, our races are filled with men and women who train that way. CrossFit is hard and it works; it gets people fit and looking good. But people who do CrossFit are not necessarily training to go out and run four or five miles, let alone thirteen. Completing a Spartan Race takes serious endurance. By the time you're doing a Spartan Beast like the one we held in Soldier Hollow, you've run, walked, and/or crawled thirteen miles. It's not a straight course, either, but rather an obstacle-filled zigzag.

I have been focused on endurance the last twenty years and that has become my passion and my refuge. I love to run what you might consider to be insanely long distances, and I'll do them with less deliberation than you probably spend picking a restaurant. You don't have to dive as deeply into endurance as I have, but you need to build some serious heart-and-lung power to complete one of our races. This is one of the most beneficial side effects of the Spartan lifestyle, because these very attributes are going to help you live a longer, fuller life too.

At rest, my now forty-seven-year-old heart beats between forty-five and fifty times a minute — half the frequency of many sedentary people. Why is this important? Whose heart do you think will wear out sooner: the one beating forty-five times a minute or the one beating ninety times a minute? So even though I'm pushing myself to crazy lengths in these endurance races, for the vast majority of my life, when I'm not racing, my heart endures less stress than the next guy's.

Spartans need to be flexible. One of the biggest problems many people face today is a lack of flexibility. One result has been an avalanche of back problems, among other things. Ignoring flexibility ties back in to instant gratification — people want beach muscles fast regardless of their long-term health and well-being. So many guys will say, "Oh, yoga, that's boring" or "That's for girls." That's nonsense and a prescription for a bad back and other injuries. Something one of my uncles said to me once sticks in my mind to this day: "It's one thing to be strong, but if you're flexible and strong, then you're really strong."

The list of fitness attributes above is a tall order, but I've found one exercise that puts it all together: the burpee, aka the squat thrust. Beginning from a standing position, drop into a squat until your hands are actually touching the ground. Without hesitation, kick your legs back to assume the up position of the pushup; do a pushup; and again without hesitation, draw your legs back into lower squat position before standing back up to starting position. From there, drop into another rep.

Think about how many great fitness elements that exercise

rolls into one. The squat alone is arguably the single best exercise known to mankind, working your entire body in a way that unleashes a cascade of natural growth hormone and other growth factors. As soon as you kick your feet back, you're in a plank, arguably the single best position for developing core strength. You also enhance cardiovascular conditioning because of the rapid-fire nature of the move when done for reps.

I think burpees are the ultimate exercise for all those reasons. In fact, if you never want to get sick again in your life, do thirty burpees a day. This works, assuming you eat healthier as well. I'm convinced that disease comes from stagnation within the body. That's why I love burpees so much, because they feel like they're lubricating all of your joints and oxygenating all of your tissues. It's a different sensation than what's produced by bench pressing or going on a rough run.

I remember when *60 Minutes* interviewed Andy and me, and they told us they were convinced that we were on to something with our emphasis on the burpee. They had first encountered it when interviewing a guy on death row who was nicknamed Big Evil. In solitary confinement Big Evil would knock out one thousand burpees a day, and the guy looked, they said, like 270 pounds of shredded steel.

As you've already read, when Spartan racers fail to complete an obstacle, they are forced to do thirty burpees. We chose burpees because it's a tough exercise that only gets harder as the race goes on; and we chose thirty reps because we determined, through trial and error, that that's the number of penalty reps that would really make you want to conquer that obstacle. If it were five burpees, people might just skip the obstacle and do the penalty reps. However, the specter of doing thirty burpees makes them think, Yeah, I really want to make this obstacle.

This book isn't a workout manual for preparing for a Spartan

Race, although we will be publishing one of those. This is about becoming fit enough to excel in your everyday life. You know by now how strongly I feel about the importance of starting each day with a workout. Not just any workout, either: military-style workouts filled with calisthenics, cardio, and other forms of conditioning. The goal is to work your entire body's musculature while elevating your heart rate and developing flexibility. Most of us don't throw big weights around the gym. Brute strength and massive muscularity isn't our goal.

What's important is setting your body in motion, and that can be done through any number of means. Swimming, for example, is another favorite activity of mine, one that works every muscle in your body, including your heart, without putting much stress on your joints. Bike riding is another great form of early morning exercise. Regardless of which exercise mode I choose, after this one hour of "suffering"—although I've come to love it—I live the rest of the day in pleasurable contrast. What's easier, exercising for one hour in the morning or being unhappy with your body twenty-four hours a day?

Researchers have found that morning exercise offers specific benefits. Exercising hard in the morning also fills a person with a sense of "I can do anything." In *Spark: The Revolutionary New Science of Exercise and the Brain*, John J. Ratey writes, "By going beyond where you thought you could, straining and stressing and lingering in that pain for even just a minute or two, you sometimes transcend into a rarefied state of mind, in which you feel like you can conquer any challenge."

One of the best training principles I've encountered goes by the acronym FITT, which stands for frequency, intensity, type of exercise, and time. Let's use an imaginary woman walking on a treadmill as an example. Her frequency is three days a week, four days a week, or however many times a week she does this. Her form of exercise is walking, not sprinting, so her intensity would be moderate. Her time is up to her. You can set those parameters as your baseline and change it from there according to the principle of progressive overload. If you're feeling good and crushing the workouts, adjust any of those variables to make them more difficult. If it's too hard, back off.

Another favorite activity of mine is high-intensity interval training. HIIT, as it's better known, alternates short bursts of furiously intense activity with short periods of downshifting. These jolts of intense activity force the body to adapt in a profoundly positive way. Researchers at the University of Bath found that sprinting as fast as you can for thirty seconds sets off a hormone blast that lasts for two hours after the sprint. You need to run as if your life depends on it, though. To paraphrase former NFL coach Denny Green, high intensity means what you think it means.

We may have evolution to thank for this effect. Those bouts of superhigh intensity exercise may mimic the body's fight-or-flight state, which would have come in handy when hunting in prehistoric times. To survive in that kill-or-be-killed situation, it would have made sense to flood your body with all the hormones needed to burn fat, build muscle, and promote brain development.

Today our survival doesn't hang in the balance of our fitness each day, so we need to find different forms of motivation. Find exercise you like to do. Exercise to increase focus or reduce stress. In the long run, our survival does indeed still hang in the balance. Dr. Ratey claims, "Paleolithic man had to walk five to ten miles an average day just to be able to eat." You probably won't be devoured by a wild animal because you were unfit to escape, but you'll be much likelier to die later from cancer, heart disease, or type 2 diabetes. The only real difference is that your death will be long and painful rather than short and painful!

The exercise you undertake doesn't even have to be to the degree that we do in preparation for Death Races and Spartan Races. It can be as simple as walking more each day. So someone living a sedentary lifestyle needs to set that goal: I want to be physically active. I don't need to exercise every day, just be physically active.

The road to success is dotted with many tempting parking places, but nothing tops the feeling of continuing down that road when you feel like giving up. Every step you take is that much closer to your goal. As Aristotle said, "We are what we repeatedly do." Imagine where you could be if you had already started. So start now. The best way to finish is to start. You can either go to bed satisfied with your efforts today or stressed with what you left for tomorrow. You can either work hard to take on the hill or never know what it is that people see at the top.

6

CHANGE YOUR DIET, CHANGE YOUR LIFE

Eat food. Not too much. Mostly plants.
— MICHAEL POLLAN

THROW OUT EVERYTHING you know about food and diet. Take it and dump it in the trash as unceremoniously as you would discard a bag of fast food remains after you leave your car. Do it before anyone sees the incriminating evidence on the car seat.

At age twenty-three, Tony Reyes was the poster child for the fast food, sedentary lifestyle that has fattened up the United States and the rest of the world. He weighed four hundred pounds and slept wearing a mask to manage sleep apnea, a condition highly correlated with obesity. Anytime the mask would slip off in the middle of the night, Tony would wake up gasping for air, certain he was about to die. Then he would sob in despair.

Tony applied to be a contestant on *The Biggest Loser* television show and made it through several rounds of casting before being eliminated. His dashed hopes made him even more despondent. A standup comedian by trade, he began to pepper his monologues with self-deprecating fat-guy jokes. The laughter didn't wash over him; it filled him with animosity for his audience and self-loathing. "Why are they all laughing and not trying to help me?" he recalls thinking. "Can't they tell I hate this life and need support to change?"

His fiancée convinced him that a television show wasn't the answer to his problems, anyway. She convinced him to sign up instead for a Spartan Sprint that was coming to Malibu, California. "When I first signed up for the race, I was scared," he recalls. "I didn't tell anyone about it because I wanted to be able to back out and quit like most of my other weight-loss attempts. I knew that elite athletes ran these races, and I didn't see anyone with my body type on any of the videos I watched."

This made him nervous, but it didn't make him quit. Everything clicked when he encountered a story on Chris Davis, a Spartan Race participant who has lost four hundred pounds over the course of his racing career. "At that moment, I knew I could do it," he says.

Working with a personal trainer, Tony began to shape up, the pounds vanishing in rapid succession. By race day, he had lost nearly one hundred pounds. Variations on this story happen every time we hold a race. Someone, perhaps many people, finally finds the motivation and accountability needed to undergo significant and sustainable weight loss. It's a remarkable thing to behold.

The American Medical Association may have voted on Tuesday, June 18, 2013, to classify obesity as a disease, but in America it's a way of life. However, being content with being overweight is the antithesis of being Spartan.

Unlike golf or baseball, you can't win a Spartan Race if you're eating junk. We designed Spartan Race to unfailingly reveal to you how efficiently your body is functioning. You don't get to rest between obstacles; there are no breaks between at bats, no timeouts, no bell ringing to signify a round's end, no stretch in the penalty box like you find in other sports. Not enough vitamins and minerals in your diet — cramps, fall behind in the race. Too many toxins floating around in your system — nausea, fall behind in the race. Too conditioned to having your stomach full — fatigue caused by low blood sugar, fall behind in the race. You can tell yourself that you are eating healthy all you want, but put it to the test, and you'll know.

Even our shortest races can suck the calories out of your body, so you need some cushion. Your body burns through your glycogen stores after two hours or so of strenuous activity, so racers must refuel every sixty to ninety minutes to avoid a crash. Try to run a Spartan Race on a Rockstar Energy Drink, which has 15.5 teaspoons of sugar in a 16-ounce can, or on some doughnuts and coffee, and you'll hit the imaginary wall before you even get to the real wall. You need deep energy reserves to a run a Spartan Race, not a quick high that will lead to a crash and failure.

Becoming a Spartan, though, is about how you eat year-round, not just on race day. Whether your goals are to lose weight, get lean, or perform better, nutrition has to be a part of your plan. Here's the one Spartan rule you must live by: "If your great grandparents didn't eat it, you probably shouldn't eat it." To me, there are a few basic reasons that so many of us lose the battle to eat healthfully:

- Great food is not always available.
- We are not completely sold that we need it, or that there is a big difference.
- If it's packaged nice and neat and it's popular, then it must be okay.

US consumers think that if a food is sitting on the shelf at the supermarket, its ingredients must have been tested by the FDA for safety, and it must be healthy. Surprise! Nice marketing and packaging and location in the right aisle don't necessarily mean that, and more than half of the chemicals added to our foods have never been FDA-tested. We have this discussion daily in our house: "Why would something packaged so well, and sold in a modern, clean supermarket, not be okay to eat? I ate it growing up, and I was fine." Well, our food supply has deteriorated.

We learn what and how to eat and drink to a large extent by observing our peers. People we admire eat and drink a certain way, so we emulate them, except maybe we're a little stricter. Unfortunately, marketing determines what's popular. Highly trained food scientists and advertising agencies are outsmarting us and preying on our tendency to fail the cookie test. Here, you need another bag of Chips Ahoy! — and you need it now.

Put ice cream next to a carrot, and what are most people going to grab first? Ice cream — and not because it's healthier or better for us. Food makers simply figured out how to sell us ice cream and a lot of it. Don't believe me? Visit Hawaii, where Spam is a delicacy and eaten daily. When food conglomerates want to sell us something, they usually succeed.

To counter this onslaught, we have to be disciplined and knowledgeable. The Spartan diet is mostly plant-based, including an abundance of vegetables and fruits. It's moderate in grains and animal food products. It eliminates processed foods, added sugars, and trans fats. Our meals are prepared from fresh foods. They don't come in a box or a wrapper.

In contrast, our society's approach to nutrition reflects our society's approach to everything: convenience above all else, no matter the long-term effects. Things like Pop-Tarts and TV dinners exist because people love to get what they want when they want it. Dissatisfied with Pillsbury's cake mix and prepared frosting, Americans demanded a product that comes already baked. And so we have premade pastries, brownies, and countless other confections. That way, we don't have to go through the outrageous trouble of actually cooking our food.

Why wait for little seeds to grow when you can give someone your money and get a mature plant in return — no gardening necessary. Take it home and plop it down wherever you like, and you've got a garden. Besides, people who plant from scratch have to worry about their plants not growing correctly, getting diseases, growing mold. All that waiting . . . most would just buy a decorative bush instead!

It's hard work for somebody to run a farm, period. Ask them to do it without pesticides or genetically modified plants, and most people won't tackle the job. I've gained nothing but dirt, leaves, some flowers, and lots of thorns from kidnapping a fully grown rose bush and installing it in my garden. I know from farming that growing from scratch is hell, but organic rotational farming has taught me in ways I never would have learned had I just *skipped to the end* like we all do.

Today, eating healthfully may be your greatest obstacle. Dietary obstacles confront us everywhere we turn in our daily lives. They appear in our urban areas and poor rural areas in "food deserts," those expanses of inhabited space lacking healthy food even for those who want it. It appears when we try to eat well in social settings while everyone else pigs out. It appears on television commercials designed to turn our kids into lifelong sugar junkies. As Samuel Johnson wrote, "The chains of habit are generally too small to be felt until they are too strong to be broken." It was true in Spartan times. It was true in Johnson's time, eighteenth-century England. It's true today.

Once we're hooked on junk food, it's hard to get unhooked, and even when people want to eat healthfully, those foods may not be accessible. Hospitals and schools, which you think would offer the best foods, often offer some of the worst.

The Spartan goes for the extra mile rather than the extra cupcake. Cars don't run on empty, so why would your body? You are what you eat, and if you eat poorly, you are more prone to injury, health complications, and possibly a shorter lifespan. A good diet will provide your body with the energy it needs to complete a successful race. It'll also make you feel better and add healthy years to your life.

Before I was lucky enough to land a job on Wall Street, I ran that pool cleaning business. To this day, I think of the swimming pool as a perfect metaphor for the human body. Each pool has a pump (heart), a filter (kidneys), water (the body is about 60 percent water), and a liner (skin). If I pumped gallons and gallons of coffee instead of water into a swimming pool every day, it would soon get sick, and the pool would turn green. The filtration system of a pool is designed to remove leaves, sand, sweat, and bacteria; it wasn't designed to remove coffee. Your body's filtration system was designed to metabolize foods found in nature, not to process the residues from laboratory-engineered substances like high-fructose corn syrup or most of the processed foods we eat. The human body is much smaller than a swimming pool, and to avoid contamination, you must eat healthy and less, drink healthy and less, sleep long enough and well enough, exercise daily, stay committed, and maintain a great attitude. A pool without that approach is not a pool you want to swim in.

When the fast-food websites offer their nutritional facts, they should change the header from NUTRITION to BRACE YOURSELF. Nutrition labels should be full of just that, NUTRITION. Not chemicals. And the fewer items on a package's ingredients list, the better. Ancient Sparta had no drive-through lanes, no golden arches beckoning to weary travelers on the interstate, no value meals, and no cheeseburgers, let alone double-doubles. The Spartan diet wasn't really a diet all, but rather part of a way of life — which is exactly how we should start thinking about food and drink. Eating was a way of fueling up to hunt and work, and meals were an opportunity for social interaction with your community.

Spartans ate to live rather than living to eat, an approach shaped by legislation put forth by the Spartan legislator Lycurgus. Two of his reforms drastically affected Spartans' sustenance. The first was a redistribution of land into plots of equal size, each large enough to grow enough barley and produce to feed its occupants. Plutarch describes the plots as producing enough to get by, but little more. This reform gave every Spartan equal access to resources. No one feasted, and no one starved.

The second reform set up common eating areas. Spartans would dine as groups of roughly fifteen in settings akin to the modern-day military mess hall. The communal nature of the meal ensured that no one starved and no one ate more than they needed. This eliminated the temptation to consume excess in private, the ancient equivalent of the modern-day midnight raid on the fridge. Each member of the mess contributed a set amount of barley meal, wine, cheese, figs, and a little extra money for meat. Everything was grown locally.

The human fighting machines that protected Sparta ran best on simple, clean foods. Plutarch described the ancient diet as consisting of a simple broth and locally grown Mediterranean produce. Spartans also ate barley bread called *maza*, presumably for carbohydrates to fuel their training, although they wouldn't have articulated it in those terms back then.

I often train on little or no food, too. I have had better athletic performances on raw fruits, vegetables, and nuts than any other diet, and I know many endurance racers who would agree. I think the idea of feasting on pasta to "carb load" before a marathon is ridiculous. Lighter eating makes for less energy expenditure. During an extended workout, I might indulge in coconut water, but that's about it; otherwise, I push through pain and discomfort. You want to give your body a break as often as you can from digesting and processing food, and you want to force your body to tap into fat storage.

This may be different from what you've heard before, or what you've done in the past, so let me elaborate. As humans, we spent the majority of our history on earth searching for food to survive. In prehistory, there was no abundance like there is today. We think we are hungry at various time during a given day, but most of us have never experienced true hunger.

I'm not suggesting you try this at home, but humans can actually live thirty to forty-five days without food if properly hydrated. In fact, I think fasting once in a while is excellent for digestive health. Imagine any engine that never gets a break; it would break down soon enough. Your gut is no different.

Doing More with Less

Spartan nutrition is all discipline and doing less with more — eating less food with a higher nutritional content. Consider these stats if you think I am being extreme:

- One in five American children between ages six and eleven are clinically obese.
- In 2000, 9 percent of US adolescents had diabetes or pre-diabetes. Now it's 23 percent.
- In Houston, Texas, 66 percent of the adults are overweight or obese.
- In 2004, no state's obesity prevalence exceeded 30 percent. From 2005 to 2007, three states did. In 2008, six states. In 2009, nine. In 2010, twelve.

On average, health care for an obese person costs $4,871 per year, whereas a normal-weight person costs $3,442 per year. Obesity isn't just a gut bomb; it's an economic time bomb.

The fattest states have the poorest, least-educated residents. Twenty percent of those living in the fifteen fattest states lack a high school diploma. The less educated people are, the less likely they are to eat healthfully, relying instead on Oreos, Cocoa Puffs, and other junk. This connection between health and wealth holds true worldwide. The wealthier countries tend to have lower obesity rates, whereas the poorer countries have the highest rates.

Unfortunately, the rest of the world is importing our diet and all the health problems that come with it. The International Diabetes Federation estimated in November 2013 that 382 million people worldwide are living with their namesake disease. One in four adults around the world has metabolic syndrome, the constellation of risk factors for diabetes and heart disease that includes obesity, low HDL, hypertension, high fasting glucose, and chronic inflammation. No coincidence that the world's population consumes roughly 165 million tons of sugar a year. Overdoing sugary foods can trigger enough chronic, low-level inflammation to speed up the aging process. The cells in your muscles and brain need glucose for energy, but too much of it coursing through your blood vessels for too long can be deadly.

Take a look around the world for more evidence we are on a collision course:

- China has the most diabetics at 92.3 million, followed by India and then the United States. Granted, China is the world's most populous nation, but that's still 9 percent of the entire country plagued with diabetes, which is shocking.
- The Middle East is a major diabetes hotspot. Check out the diabetes prevalence in these member nations: Kuwait, 23.9 percent; Saudi Arabia, 23.4 percent; Qatar, 23.3 percent; and Bahrain, 22.4 percent.

- Mexico is now the developed world's fattest nation, excluding a few small island nations in the Pacific. Diabetes kills as many people there in one year as the drug wars kill in six.
- Aboriginal populations are the hardest hit once they forsake their traditional ways and adopt a more Western diet and lifestyle. For example, the people of Samoa were just fine until they stopped working for their food. Now two-thirds of urban Samoans are obese. Similarly, the Pima Indians' diabetes rates increase by a factor of five after they began living in a more Western fashion.

In the United States alone, 160,000 fast-food restaurants serve 50 million people daily, ringing up $110 billion in annual sales. Every day, one in four Americans eats fast food. At the same time, there has been a decline in manual-labor jobs and an increase in service-sector jobs. So we eat more and sit more, a toxic brew. The swimming pool is being filled daily with processed foods, and the pump and filter is running a lot less frequently — a deadly combination.

Lower-income families had a lot more free time in 1999 than they did in 1965, but nearly all that time in 1999 was spent watching television. This is because TVs had become cheaper. Low-income families, which tend to have less education and, consequently, less knowledge of how to eat right, and who can suddenly afford a TV set, tend to become obese because they eat poorly and sit for long periods.

Combine too many calories + not enough physical activity = type 2 diabetes. Physicist and geneticist James Neel argues that type 2 diabetes is the body's natural reaction to an increase in readily available calories. It makes sense. Hunter-gatherers — our ancestors of long ago — had to be able to go for long periods under intense stress, much like that of an adventure race. So, millions of years ago, their body adapted. "Our hunter-gatherer ancestors would have found the idea of exercise for exercise's sake ludicrous," wrote Ellen Ruppel Shell in *The Hungry Gene*. That's because life for them was about finding and saving calories.

Fast forward to thousands of years ago and the advent of agriculture. Confronted by an abundance of carbohydrates, the finely tuned metabolic system of the human body couldn't handle it. Ancient people started getting cavities when they ate all the starchy foods that were being farmed. Now, with an even greater abundance of cheap starch and sugar thanks to the Industrial Revolution, the human body becomes very confused — and that confusion leads to obesity and type 2 diabetes, the disease of the couch.

In the Paleolithic period, people died primarily as the result of bodily trauma — either through childbirth, war with neighboring tribes, or by hunting accidents. ("I thought he was the moose!") After humans started domesticating animals, infectious diseases that were contracted by hanging around farm animals — such as smallpox, measles, and tuberculosis — became the main cause of death. Nowadays, armed with vaccines and antibiotics, we struggle with noncommunicable diseases like obesity. It seems that our greatest health problems are products of society, and hence our own creation. We've invented ways to slowly kill ourselves!

I think the calorie is the wrong unit of measure for most of us to use. It doesn't mean anything to most people, and it clearly won't stop us from overeating the wrong foods. We often say around the Spartan offices that we should measure our food in burpees rather than calories. It's a punishing exercise we use in our races, and if eating bad food resulted in immediate punishment, people might alter their behavior.

We've created a formula to convert foods to burpees. For example, a McDonald's large fry is more than 500 burpees. Depending on brand, a beer could be 150 burpees. This kind of penalty can help combat the food marketers and scientists. Who wants to do 500 burpees?

You can't wish for a fit body. You have to go get it. You have to be willing to eat and exercise your way there. You used to be able to walk into a food store, make your way around the perimeter, check out, and leave. Now we have fifty aisles loaded with items that are basically chemistry experiments. There are a few healthy cereals and breads down there, but for the most part it's junk in the center aisles. One reason we're a nation of fast-food zombies is that not nearly enough people ever learn how to cook, let alone healthfully. And even if they did, who has the time?

Do you realize that you'd have to eat to eat 130 strawberries to equal the 520 calories in one McDonald's Quarter Pounder with Cheese? That you'd need to eat three whole oranges to equal the amount of sugar in one glass of orange juice? Of course we have an obesity pandemic! It was inevitable, given how we've feasted on fast food and swilled liquid sugar for half a century.

Even when fast-food chains attempt to incorporate fruit into their menu, they take a healthy-sounding item and turn it into a gut bomb. While blueberries are a Spartan-approved food choice, the 22-ounce McCafé Blueberry Pomegranate Smoothie contains 17.5 teaspoons of sugar. Bananas are healthy but not when they're caramel-coated. Denny's Banana Caramel French Toast Skillet has 87 grams of sugar! The Dairy Queen Kid's Strawberry Banana Smoothie contains nearly 10 teaspoons of sugar, more than a kid should consume all day.

Baked goods are another huge contributor to runaway obesity rates. If you want to lose the muffin top, get rid of the doughnuts, croissants, and bagels! Lift weights, not cake. As Jack LaLanne said, "The only good part of a doughnut is the hole in the middle."

Sugar is an enemy of the body and one of the substances it

finds the most addictive. It causes tooth decay, leads to chronic inflammation, increases insulin levels in the body, contributes to the onset of type 2 diabetes, and has even been linked to several deadly cancers. That's just for starters. We all know it contributes to obesity and heart disease.

Foods with added sugars tend to be high in calories and low in vitamins and minerals. Junk food fare also leaves you shortchanged when it comes to fiber. A high-fiber diet helps you control your blood sugar, feel fuller for longer, and better manage your weight. You need at least fourteen grams of fiber for every one thousand calories you take in. Fiber helps with weight loss, colon health, and glycemic (blood sugar) control.

Instead, we turn fruit into fruit juice, we transform water into carbonated soda, and our body never knows what hit it because all these liquid calories flood past our satiety sensors in ways that whole foods can't. Don't believe it? Try eating as much salad as you want one day, and see if you overeat. Food companies know this when they are marketing to us. According to a University of North Carolina study, the average American drinks 450 liquid calories a day and 53 gallons of soft drinks per year. On a typical day, four out of five children and two out of three adults drink sugar-sweetened beverages, which their bodies cannot handle day in, day out.

Kids crave sugar and their parents give it to them, even when they don't know they're doing it. Flavored yogurt, salad dressings, breads, sauces and marinades, tomato sauce, peanut butter, cereals — all are frequently sweetened with sugar during processing, unbeknownst to many of the people consuming them. Most bottles of ketchup are 25 percent sugar! This is not a vegetable.

My mother used to tell my sister and me that sugar is a drug, but we couldn't believe it. Why would it be in everything we eat, and why were all the other kids getting to eat it? Well, researchers at Princeton University have studied the effects of sugar on the brain chemistry of rats, and what they've found is that their subjects exhibit all the effects of heroin addiction. Sugar does this by triggering the release of the feel-good chemical dopamine in the section of the brain normally associated with addictive behaviors. The dopamine release produces a druglike high. Yet the brain adapts. So it takes more of the substance — in this case, sugar — to produce the same effect. This makes it a great addition to any food — if you are in the business of selling food.

According to the lead researcher in the Princeton study, a psychologist named Bart Hoebel, "Our evidence from an animal model suggests that bingeing on sugar can act in the brain in ways very similar to drugs of abuse."

Lessening the sugar stimulation only makes the body want more dopamine. Remove the substance altogether, and the sugar abuser experiences physical and psychological withdrawal symptoms. The body is addicted. Twinkies aren't classified as a controlled substance, but for the glucose intolerant, perhaps they should be.

Breaking the cycle means avoiding blood-sugar crashes. To do this, you need to eat protein, healthy fats (monounsaturated and polyunsaturated), and fibrous vegetables for breakfast, a meal normally stocked with simple sugars and other fast-acting carbohydrates. A carb that is at least 20 percent fiber is a quality source. Those are increasingly the exception to what people consume.

Read your food labels! Know the code names that are used to disguise sugar on food labels: dextrose/maltodextrin, fructose, fruit juice concentrate, glucose, high-fructose corn syrup, honey, maple syrup, molasses, sucrose, and xylose. Avoid the foods whose packages list them. Better yet, switch from packaged to whole foods. Look at the label where it says "sugars" and divide those grams by four to get teaspoons, a more visual measure. So the forty grams in a can of soda equals ten teaspoons. Do we really need to drink ten teaspoons of sugar? Think fruit juice is better? Not by much.

Exercise daily, which not only helps usher sugar out of your bloodstream but also produces good-vibe brain chemicals of its own called endorphins. You want to get a runner's high, not a sugar high.

Food should be fuel for your workouts, not medication for your moods. Many people try to cheer themselves up by giving themselves treats. It's an enticing idea. You're feeling sad so you treat yourself to your favorite movie or your favorite snack as a means of feeling better and more comfortable. Get those ideas out of your head. Research shows that this doesn't work, which should not surprise us at all. To me, it looks like just another way of taking the cookie now. What you really ought to do is find a way to reassert your ability to achieve. When you're feeling down, the easy thing to do is to sit and wallow in self-pity. But you've got to pull yourself together. Depression is one of the most grueling cookie tests because every moment is a choice either to stay the same or seek change.

Transformation Trigger Point

Andi Hardy, who is now a member of the Spartan Pro Team, knows this feeling all too well. She fell out of shape and packed on pound after pound until one day, she woke up and couldn't take it anymore. "I had tipped the scale to a number that totally disgusted me," she recalls. "It wasn't just the number that glared at me from that little square thing on the floor beneath my feet; it was the discomfort of my clothes, the zippers that required an extra tug, the buttons that pulled a little too far to the side of the buttonholes and the tire that wobbled around my middle."

As happens with so many people, one attempt at weight loss after another failed. Nothing seemed to work. "Each attempt ended with a big bowl of ice cream topped with peanut butter and chocolate syrup," she says. "Not this time, this was it; I had had it with myself."

She found an online weight-loss program that she liked and started logging her meals and working out regularly. She will be the first to admit that she often felt miserable and deprived as she watched friends devour her favorite foods while she ate raw vegetables. But something amazing was happening too. The weight that had become so burdensome began to decrease. Emboldened by her progress, she entered a triathlon, finishing in the top ten in her age group among more than one hundred.

Later she did an obstacle race, and then heard about the Spartan Race, which she entered as well. "Training for that first Spartan Race was not easy either," she recalls. "I knew that I had to train hard, but also really had to watch what I put into my body. I kept learning about food and portions."

Today, she's a new woman. A Spartan woman. "I'm finally comfortable in my skin," she says. "I am not the skinniest woman, nor do I have the body of a model, but I wear what I want and race in a skimpy outfit and don't feel embarrassed by my skin — or by what used to jiggle around under it."

The pain, the brokenness that led to Andi's downward spiral is happening everywhere. How did we get into this metabolic mess in the first place? We not only have things backward when it comes to food consumption, but also when it comes to food production. Poor food starts with poor food production. Farming became industrialized around the time of the world wars to feed a lot of people fast. We needed to grow food faster, bigger, and cheaper, and in the process, farming got broken.

But there is a new trend to bring farming and food production back to the way it was meant to be done. Some small farms around the country are starting to rotate the animals and plants and their byproducts the way nature would. They are getting away from mass-production farming that smells like septic waste when you drive by it. We are starting to learn that it is not healthy to pack thousands of animals into a small barn. Unfortunately, only a small group of people are committed to organic rotational farming, but it's gaining momentum and has even made its way into supplying large companies such as Whole Foods. Even a fast-food company like Chipotle is trying to do it better. If we know all this, why isn't it changing faster? The issue is patience, and if you have it, you are certainly rewarded.

As our society follows the cosmopolitan trends of each week, many people are still uncertain when it comes to eating organic. After all, the US government certified organic food only beginning about six and a half years ago. While the health advantages of organic foods are hotly debated, a systematic review in a September 2012 issue of *Annals of Internal Medicine* found that "organic foods may reduce exposure to pesticide residues and antibiotic-resistant bacteria." While it will take several more years for data to be gathered, many people are not waiting. They're pursuing this lifestyle today. Don't rely on the medical journals — just come visit our farm in Vermont, and you'll see what I'm talking about. You'll agree, I'm hoping, that all of our food should come from local, organic, rotational grazing farms.

According to an article in the *Atlantic,* the earth essentially cannot produce more food than it does now. With a projected world population of nine billion people in 2050, the only hope for feeding the human race is a departure from meat- and dairy-based diets among the wealthier nations of the world in favor of a more sustainable, primarily vegetarian lifestyle. The calories in grains that could be used to support human life are largely lost in the bodies of cows and other livestock. The meat that we finally consume from these animals has only a fraction of the calories that the original grains had.

Some opponents of organic farming argue that organic crops have a low yield and that farmers were forced to use pesticides and other chemicals to increase their yield and feed a growing population. "Till the entire population can be fed," says T. N. Manjunath of Agri Biotechnology, "there is no way one can ban the use of chemicals and pesticides." We need a high yield of crops like corn so that we can feed our animals and get meat — but if we stopped eating so much meat, the demand for certain grains would decrease significantly.

The terms we use to describe organic and conventional farming are backwards. We call industrialized farming "conventional" despite the fact that it's a recent phenomenon. Organic farming has effectively been around for thousands of years.

Given the Spartan Race emphasis on healthy nutrition, it may come as no surprise that we're big believers in natural farming and organic food and critics of agribusiness and processed foods. I live on an organic farm and consider myself a working farmer when I'm not running Spartan Race. Working the soil is peaceful. After all, the soil is where we come from and where we go when this is over. Toiling in it feels like being home to me. Making food from seeds is incredibly satisfying.

At the Spartan Race, our approach to nutrition supplies the human body's need for a steady supply of fresh fruits and vegetables. Science has proven that consuming plenty of fruits and vegetables protects against chronic disease in numerous ways. Given that many of these diseases are growing more like epidemics rather than chronic conditions, you might assume that we're falling short with our fruits and veggie intake. Indeed we are: The US government recommendation calls for 9 servings of either/or per day; the average American manages only 3.6 servings, a little more than a third of the daily requirement. In the absence of these essential nutrients, diseases, rather than good health, can gain the upper hand.

Fruits and vegetables are packed with vitamins, minerals, healthy plant chemicals, and fiber. Mother nature, as it turns out, is a pretty adept chemist. You may have heard terms like *phenolics*, *flavonoids*, and *carotenoids*, but you may not know what they mean. Well, they're all phytochemicals — but *phyto* just means plant. So they're chemicals found in edible plants. Different fruits and veggies are higher or lower in different plant chemicals, but they all have their unique profile and combinations.

Many of these vital nutrients are now available in tablet form. Nothing against dietary supplements, but the Spartan way is to find them in whole foods. Here are some that we always try to include in our weekly diet:

- Berries: Blueberries, raspberries, and strawberries are superfoods with antioxidant, anticancer, antimicrobial, anti-inflammatory, and anti-nerve-degeneration compounds. They're rich in what are called *polyphenols*, which are plant substances that help slow the aging process, protecting your mind and body. The compound that makes blueberries blue, a polyphenol called anthocyanin, also helps relax your blood vessels, among other benefits. Blueberries even contain resveratrol, the antiaging compound best known for its presence in red wine.

- Apples: One reason an apple a day keeps the doc away is that each medium-sized one contains four grams of soluble fiber, which helps to steady blood sugar. Steady blood sugar helps your arteries stay healthy and keeps hunger pangs at bay. Apples are also rich sources of cancer-fighting antioxidants, many of which reside in the peel — one more reason to eat the whole fruit and skip the apple juice.

- Vegetables: I'm going to single out a few vegetables below, but vegetables as an entire class of food are Spartan approved. You can buy them whole or even precut if you want to save time.

Women may be able to cut breast cancer risk by 15 to 20 percent by eating kale, spinach, tomatoes, carrots, bell peppers, and so on. Broccoli is loaded with vitamins, glucosinolates, phenolic compounds, and dietary essential minerals. These nutrients protect against a laundry list of health threats, including cancer.

- Almonds: Monounsaturated fat, fiber, α-tocopherol, magnesium, copper, phytonutrients — all are found in relative abundance in this nutrient-dense and satiating snack. No wonder they lower heart risks.

- Avocado: This is actually a fruit, and it's one of the healthiest foods you can consume, offering potential health benefits against inflammation and cancer cell growth. Power up your smoothies or salads with one of the healthiest fatty foods out there!

- Edamame: This version of the soybean is as addictive a snack as popcorn, yet it's full of protein, fiber, and phytochemicals. Studies have found that edamame may have antidiabetic effects, not surprising given their high fiber content.

- Eggs: This is a great protein source for any athlete or fitness enthusiast. Only remove the yolks if you want to cut some calories; otherwise, they contain important nutrients.

- Quinoa: This superfood is a complete nonmeat protein. An ancient grain, it is one of your most healthy choices and great for farming. The world would be a healthier and less stressed planet if we grew more quinoa and raised less livestock on our farms.

- Garlic: We had four Slovakians working for us on our farm in Vermont, and they would toil nonstop for twelve hours a day. Every day, these four guys would eat raw garlic. They had done this, they said, their entire lives. Because they worked so hard and sweated to so much, the garlic would rise from their pores like steam escaping from a manhole cover. The reverse works as well, with garlic entering pores in the skin. These same guys told me that some people would put raw garlic in their socks before going to bed at night.

As it turns out, when scientists put raw garlic in a petri dish, it kills everything harmful in sight. Garlic contains tons of antioxidants. Voodoo witch doctors wore garlic around their neck because they believed it would kill evil spirits that manifested themselves as sickness. Today, researchers have identified a key compound in garlic, called allicin, whose many health benefits include protecting against both of America's two biggest killers: heart disease and cancer. Cooking with garlic seems to negate or at least reduce many of these health benefits, however. Consume it raw instead.

Water is also critically important for general health and Spartan racing. Studies find that most people drink roughly the same amount of liquid each day. So as you drink more water, you drink fewer sodas.

A study of longevity in humans identified several areas in America where life expectancy exceeded the norm. These areas, which scientists call blue zones, were also found to have high populations of Seventh-Day Adventists. I'm not suggesting we all become Adventists, but we might learn something here. It turns out that the traditional lifestyle and diet of Adventists tends to increase lifespan by several years. The Adventist lifestyle consists, broadly speaking, of vegetarianism, an abstinence from tobacco products, a frequent consumption of nuts, a commitment to exercise, and maintaining a "normal body weight." Dan Buettner, author of the book that explores the blue-zone phenomenon, recommends nine strategies for improving overall health:

1. Practice physical movement as much as possible.
2. Find a sense of lasting purpose.
3. Reduce stress.
4. "80 percent rule"— Eat only to 80 percent satisfaction.
5. Eat less meat and more "beans, lentils, and nuts."
6. Drink a reasonable amount of alcohol every day.
7. Find a strong community — and stay there.
8. Nurture family relationships.
9. Develop relationships that support your values.

Every one of these strategies is also a Spartan strategy. I even like the fact that he places exercise first, where it belongs. There are six components to fitness: cardiovascular fitness, muscular strength, muscle endurance, flexibility, body composition, and nutrition. Nutrition is more important than nearly 20 percent of the equation, though. To me, being fit is 50 percent nutrition, 50 percent hard work. You can work out all you want, but if you eat crap food, you're going to look and feel like crap. Nutrition is so important to your overall performance; without proper fuel, how can you possibly expect your body to perform well?

Eating clean today is for tomorrow. Clean food helps you recover from hard work and high stress alike. Spartan Race wants to lead the charge in crushing obesity. C'mon, do we really need a physician to treat obesity? Why not nip it in the bud before it gets to that point? I want to rip seventy-eight million people off of their couches and get them to follow the Spartan lifestyle.

7

MOVING PAST MOUNTAINS

Opportunity is missed by most people because it is dressed in overalls and looks like work.

— THOMAS EDISON

W E DON'T BUILD a Spartan Race on an entirely flat surface for many reasons. Most of all, that's not fun and makes it hard to test your limits. Almost everyone is drawn to climb a hill, even if it's just to see a nice view. Heart-pumping hills are an important part of any Spartan course. Some hills are steeper and more taxing than others, but the climbs are always there, daring you to conquer them, sometimes almost mocking you. You can practice all you want on a treadmill by setting a steep incline, but running up a mountain can't be replicated in the gym. Even seasoned athletes will hit these rises hard, only to slow to a walk and then stop altogether, out of gas. We have seen all levels of athletes stopped in their tracks by Spartan Race terrain.

Life is much the same way. Poor genetics are a mountain. School is a mountain. Heartbreak is a mountain. Divorce is a mountain. Obesity is a mountain. Layoffs are a mountain. A blown disc in your spine is a mountain. The death of parents is a mountain. Chemotherapy is a mountain. Multiple sclerosis is a mountain. They come at us one after the other. Some seduce us slowly, some scare the shit out of us immediately, but they never stop coming. That's why every Spartan race demands that you climb hills and overcome obstacles — because life does this to each of us.

The rejection I received when I first applied to Cornell stunned me, but failures like that are important in life, even if you don't realize it at the time. They humble us. They teach us lessons. Without that failure, I wouldn't have worked my ass off for the next two years doing whatever I could to gain entry to Cornell. Failure can be your greatest asset if you use it to move forward and progress. It can be an incredible motivator, and the sooner a person learns that in life, the further that person can go.

On the flip side, quitting a race brings instant relief. When you slow down, step off the course, crawl into bed, and give in, it actually feels awesome for a few hours. It's the same momentary relief you get from quitting a difficult job or a challenging relationship. Whew! you say to yourself. But that failure may sting for years to come. In contrast, unrelenting persistence gets you to the finish line and everything that the finish line represents. Learn to enjoy life by *doing,* and then you'll not only seize every day, but you will also be happy and productive during the challenging parts of your day and life.

"Good" failures humble us yet teach us valuable lessons. Let's say you prepared insanely well for a life event, but you could never have anticipated what would come your way. How do you make it through? Think of the Olympic hopeful who trains their whole life and then has a bad day in the Olympic trials. Attitude in life is everything. With the right attitude, you can climb all those mountains even when the terrain is brutal.

Can attitude be taught? Based on my experience watching countless people succeed only by challenging themselves, I believe the answer is yes. The way to improve your attitude is to push through adversity. Once you have seen the dark side, you push through until that dark phase comes to an end, and everything after that appears brighter, more hopeful. I have a saying I use whenever I'm uncomfortable: "It could be worse. I could be freezing in Alaska or surrounded by sharks." Whatever is bothering you in that moment suddenly doesn't seem so bad. This too shall pass.

Take, for example, a woman who was morbidly obese. Blair Christie was there as recently as 2009, sitting on the couch, eating junk, getting fat, and growing more depressed. "I was just shy of three hundred pounds and really struggling with my self-image. I could not even bend over to tie my shoelaces without getting winded. How could I consider doing a Spartan Race?"

Like many people, she had to hit rock bottom; she had to crawl out of the ravine before she could even see the mountain. But with the encouragement of friends helping her along when her own enthusiasm flagged, she took control over her life. Over three and a half years, she lost 120 pounds. She has run a half marathon, a full marathon, and become a certified Tae Bo instructor, allowing her to help others achieve the same sort of weight-loss success that she has. She has also become a Spartan Racer. "I currently weigh less than I did in fourth grade!"

"These races have challenged me to a whole new level of fitness," she says. "I'm thankful that I know that you don't get any better if you don't push yourself outside of your comfort zone. I am excited about always getting better and stronger. I cannot lie and say that I am not nervous about race day, but what a sweet victory when I cross the finish line!"

Mountains are more than just a metaphor, though. When you're trekking or running progressively higher, your lungs suck larger and larger amounts of air. The lactic acid burns in your hamstrings and your quads feel like they're on fire. Sweat pours out of you, and your mind sometimes starts playing tricks on you. There's no easy way out, no shortcut, no conveyor belt you can hop on at the airport because you can't carry a piece of luggage from the security checkpoint to the gate. The mountain doesn't give a shit why you slacked on your workouts the past nine months. The mountain wants to kick your ass, not help you on your way. Mountains keep the weak away from whatever lies on the other side of them.

When I think about mountains as an obstacle, perhaps the defining one, I'm reminded of the Spartan Beast held in Vermont in November 2011. A racer named Rose Marie Jarry finished fourth among all women who entered the race. While an experienced racer, she entered on impulse and lacked her normal preparation. There's a fine line between healthy impulsiveness and hubris, and she was straddling it. Much of the race wound steeply through mountain passes, and she passed me with a backward-looking grin during the first hours of the race, so you know she was truckin' along pretty well. But, at the two-and-a-half-hour mark, I caught up to her. She was stuck in the mountains, a fifty-pound sack on her back. She had struggled through this rocky pass for fifty minutes, and the bag that was her burden was falling apart at the seams.

The mountain passage had become so tight that she blocked our path, so I gently pushed on the disintegrating sack she was carrying to help her get moving again.

"Thanks, Joe," she said. "This mountain really wants to kick my ass today, and this sack isn't helping matters."

The sack was an important and telling addition. Today, climbing is a sport or a hobby for many people, but if it's a means of exploration, you carry heavy objects with you to survive. They slow you down, but you need them. You don't reach the top then get helicoptered down to a lodge to celebrate.

"After that I told myself I was going to do some weights for more upper body strength, to avoid repeating the same irritating situation," she said afterward. "Also, I vowed to work on leg conditioning because those steep hills caused my quads to burn for ten days after the race. I was walking like I needed a set of crutches."

Rose Marie climbed the mountain.

Grit Is Soul Food

There's strength, and then there's Spartan strength, the ability to commit to working for a long period of time without any concrete evidence that it will pay off—doing it because you want to, not because you have to. Mahatma Gandhi's peaceful campaign for Indian sovereignty required Spartan strength, because there were many times when it looked like it was going nowhere. India still hadn't gained independence from Britain when Gandhi died—he never saw the two cookies. But still he persevered for his entire life.

Spartan strength relates to a term I discussed earlier: grit, an innate trait that nonetheless can become ingrained through dedication and application. Grit refers to an indefatigable will to overcome obstacles, like that steep mountain pass that nearly brought Rose Marie to her knees. Think of it this way:

- Spartan strength is the determination that arises out of true commitment.
- Grit is the assertion and application of will to fulfill that commitment.

Spartan strength emerges out of a psychic alignment to get something done. That alignment is determined and unbreakable: this is just what is going to be. Grit emerges out of the force of will that manifests action. Grit is execution. Grit actually gets shit done.

Combine the two and greatness can emerge: the Edmund Hillarys who climb to the top of Mount Everest, the Magellans who die sailing around the world. Grit isn't always applied physically, either. It's the Edisons who perfect a light bulb design after thousands of failed attempts.

Spartan strength and grit are what we're looking for in the

Death Race and in the Spartan Race. We've determined that they're
the most important factors in personal success. To succeed at life
we must be able to do that which sucks: working late on a weekend
in order to meet a deadline; doing what your boss tells you to do
even if you don't agree with it; studying for days to score high on
midterms. These activities are not fun — they suck — but you have
to do them in order to succeed. If you approach life the right way,
you can turn that which, from the outside, looks like it will suck or
be miserable into something fun to overcome.

We learn to be gritty, or we learn not to be gritty. The alarm
goes off at 5:00 A.M. — what do you do? Believe it or not, our success in life often hangs in the balance. If we go through life hitting
the snooze button, our chances for success plunge. We are dramati-
cally decreasing our odds of success in life. When successful execu-
tives are studied, one of the basic common denominators found is
that they all wake up early and work out. None of them are hitting
snooze. They all know that if you snooze, you lose.

Developing grit is easier said than done, but there are specific
strategies to do so, which include:

1. Making a commitment, one that will make life better for you
   and for those around you.
2. Determining what kinds of bullshit usually gets in the way of
   your fulfilling said commitment.
3. Learning how to recognize the bullshit when it sneaks up on
   you and telling it to go away by focusing solely on the task at
   hand.
4. Executing the task at hand as if your ass is on fire.
5. Recommitting and doing it all again!

Make sure the goal in question matters. Otherwise you'll think,
Why did I want to do this in the first place? People are motivated

to complete the Spartan Trifecta because self-esteem is vital to their survival and essential to their happiness in life. If someone joins the "300 Burpees Club"—a club for anyone who has completed three hundred burpees in a row—they can associate themselves in their own minds with the other individuals who have joined that elite group.

To achieve a new goal, it helps to have practice in achieving other unpleasant goals. This provides confidence that you can achieve whatever you put your mind to—to convince you that you have grit. Religion often works this way. Continuing the motions of belief as you work out issues can help you transcend your doubt and achieve that which you didn't think you could. This is a powerful tool.

Many young people haven't developed grit because they have never been truly motivated to accomplish anything. Their survival never depended on it, certainly not in the way it did for those young Spartan warriors when they were cast out in the wilderness alone to survive or perish. This is why they may lose interest and never make it that far. Today I was walking in the mountains of Vermont with three of my kids, ages four to seven, and near the four-hour mark, they started complaining. I thought, if they normally did eight hours a day, this would be a piece of cake. If all kids did eight hours a day, they would most likely learn over time that pain goes away, that time passes and they get through it, all on the way to becoming Spartan strong.

The mere act of signing up for a Spartan Race is an initial spark of Spartan strength and grit. The aspiration to join a Spartan Race is similar to the feeling we get watching a movie about becoming a soldier or athlete, or a movie like *Die Hard*, where an ordinary guy becomes a hero. "Boy, I can see myself doing that. I could do it if I had to. That'd be cool!"

The trick with Spartan Race is that you *can* do it. It's easy to make this commitment, because you are simply saying yes! Then, because you are often in a group setting when engaging with Spartan, you have to develop grit, because the team is relying on you. You don't want to let them down, you don't want to let me down, and eventually, you don't want to let yourself down.

So you actually don't have the right amount of grit right off the bat. Grit is developed in you like a muscle!

Get the Balance Right

In ancient Greece, a group called the Stoics drew a hard line between what people can and cannot change. In contrast to our "everybody gets a trophy" society, the Stoics did not believe that human beings could be anything they wanted to be. In that culture, people were born into social classes they couldn't transcend. It's not tragic; that's just the way it was. But the Stoics did believe that all human beings had control over their beliefs, efforts, desires, and actions. While a person was pretty much stuck in his social rank, body, and responsibilities, he still had his will, with which, as the ancient Greek philosopher Epictetus says, he could pursue and attain great things.

Spartan discipline means chucking everything that "weighs down the boat." My health is a priority for me, so when I look for food to eat I ask myself, "Will this steak make the boat go faster? Will it improve my health?" If not, then it's not a difficult decision—I won't eat it. But as an athlete, I'm well aware that certain foods work better at certain times than others. A piece of fruit eaten thirty minutes before an endurance event will be metabolized much differently than the same food consumed ten minutes before bed. Protein consumed post-workout will be more effective than protein consumed at some other time, because your body is primed for protein synthesis and post-workout muscle growth.

These decisions are all about priorities, and the Spartan life involves nothing if not setting priorities. Epictetus summed it up perfectly: "Aiming therefore at such great things, remember that you must not allow yourself to be carried, even with a slight tendency, towards the attainment of lesser things. Instead, you must entirely quit some things and for the present postpone the rest." Great things in this case are those that are immeasurably important to you.

Discipline involves postponing that which you'd really like to do but which surely won't help you in the long run. Without discipline, you won't reach your goals except by pure happenstance. Without the resolve to avoid those things that slow you down, trip you up, and make you feel awful the next day, it's impossible to speed up, to keep walking, or to be healthy.

Pain is inevitable in the world of Spartan racing. In training or on racing days, we stub a toe, trip on a root, jam a finger, cramp up, even break a bone — the list goes on. I've had my eyelids freeze shut during endurance races. We eat something that doesn't sit right with our stomach. We feel pain when we exercise. Our muscles seize up, our tendons get tight, we break the lactic acid threshold and feel our bodies crying *"Stop!"* with every vein and every bone. It's a rare day that ends without a ding or two.

Pain serves a purpose, though. It keeps us from touching hot stoves, from stabbing ourselves with forks when we eat, from biting our tongues off, and from otherwise injuring ourselves. If we didn't know pain, we would never be satisfied with simple pleasures such as eating, resting, and living.

People experience each day from certain frames of reference, a phrase I use a lot in this book. These frames have lows, normals, and highs, which might loosely correspond to pain, normal, and pleasure. Using our conscious and subconscious memory, we evaluate everything that happens to us according to what has already happened, according to the lows and highs that we have experienced. The normal level always falls between the other two. That said, in order to believe that what's happening right now is good, it has to be equal to or higher than your normal level. Otherwise you're left wanting.

Rites of Passage

I apply this theory in what I like to call "Rites of Passage." These might involve a ten-hour bike ride through the mountains in the dark, an ultramarathon, or an eight-day trek through Alaskan wilderness without rest. You're probably asking yourself why I willingly put myself through this hell. I must enjoy suffering, right? Well, yes and no. Nobody likes to suffer. After all, you're not suffering if you like it. I don't enjoy the second half of an ultra, because then I'm suffering. But when the suffering ends, when the proverbial storm clears and you see the sun, when you cross the finish line at the Iditarod and gulp down those four ounces of water from a flimsy plastic cup — that's when you realize how good it feels not to suffer. Nothing tops the feeling of continuing when you feel like giving up. It changes everything, because it recalibrates your frame of reference.

Normal is what you make it. Normal for a kid who walks to and from school every day is different from normal for a kid driven to and from school in a BMW every day. Normal is different for an Eskimo living in an igloo than it is for someone growing up in a Beverly Hills mansion. Our mind creates limits around what is "normal." It's not normal to run continuously for twenty-four hours. It's not possible. . . . Says who? What if you were tracking big game, and it was your only chance of survival?

Only once you've learned to deal with pain can you demonstrate extraordinary strength. At the Fiji Eco Challenge in 2005 I got lost, and a small group of Fijian boys led me and a few other endurance athletes through the Fiji interior, a dense jungle with no roads. I was wearing biking shoes because my running footwear had been stolen. It took us five hours of making our way through incredibly dense vegetation, listening to strange sounds that I assume were exotic animals, but these kids ultimately walked us to the next village. Their machetes cut through the high immovable brush like an American lawnmower takes down grass. They skipped through rivers, hopped over hills, and climbed up muddy, slippery mountain trails without the proper shoes I always thought we needed. In fact, they had no shoes.

I gave their leader my fancy GPS adventure-racing watch as a way to say thank-you, and then months later I sent him rugby uniforms for his team. That boy who led us to safety wasn't much older than my seven-year-old son Jack, but for him, walking barefoot through a jungle wielding a machete was a common occurrence.

The ability to tap into extraordinary strength based on need resides in all of us. And, yet, we don't know how to call it up under regular circumstances. But these examples exist, so we know it's possible. We can impose limits on ourselves or we can create unlimited extraordinary experiences.

Learn to Dose Your Pain

Here's a quick checklist for internalizing the process of the "dosing of pain," the proper management of time, and the fast decision-making of the Rule of Upside Downside.

1. Realize that time is the most precious asset we have.
2. Once you truly understand this, you learn how to make sure you don't waste any. All of your time is used in a way that maximizes the achievement of your goals.

3. Understand that time passes whether we like it or not. Every second another second is gone. When you truly understand that, it helps you in those moments when you're uncomfortable. You know you can handle it if it's for a greater good.

4. Why does quick decision making matter here? You don't want to waste more time than required in making decisions. This will sound harsh but none of us know if we will be here one minute from now. If you understand that, you won't want to waste time being unproductive. If you can make accurate decisions quickly, you have time to enjoy the fruits of those decisions.

I always try to look at the upside versus the downside of each decision. You should value:

- Health first
- Family second
- Business third
- Fun fourth

Most people have these priorities upside down, whereas I make my decisions based on that hierarchy. If I'm stuck in the lobby of a hotel for an hour waiting for someone, sure, it might be fun to watch TV. Instead, I might decide to stretch out while sitting — without disturbing other guests — to maximize my time and place my health before the fun of watching TV.

Really understanding time is what has helped me push through numerous events and challenges over the years. While in some sense time is the enemy, it also allows you to break pain down and dole it out in the same way you're accustomed to delivering rewards.

The way to get through anything mentally painful is to take it a little at a time. The mind can't handle dealing with a massive iceberg of pain in front of it, but it can deal with short nuggets that will come to an end. So instead of thinking, Ugh, I've got twenty-four miles to go, focus on making it to the next telephone pole in the distance. Whether you're running twenty or one hundred and twenty miles at a time, the distance has to be tackled mentally and physically one mile at a time. The ability to compartmentalize pain into these small bite sizes is key.

In prehistory, humans would track their prey and wear them out, hunting them till they were exhausted. The ability to "lock on" to a bigger goal is valuable, and it's easier when you are in the hunt. That is why working out or racing against competition is so much more powerful — because you are in the hunt. As humans we are uniquely developed to do this — track prey for days, even though they're far faster than we are. It's the classic tortoise and hare metaphor. Many animals are faster, but we win in the end.

I'll trudge through endurance events for days on end, but I'll make trivial and life-changing decisions alike on a dime. While this may seem contradictory, it reflects another aspect of the Spartan-ness. We are decisive, but we're more than that. We are decisive *fast*. To "Spartan up!" you must decide things quickly. Wait too long, and you'll lose. If you *are* losing, lose fast, get it over with, move over, and start winning. It's a lesson I learned on Wall Street many times: sometimes you need to cut your losses quickly so you're not totally fucked later on.

I've been decisive and fast in all facets of my life, even my relationship with my wife. I met Courtney at a relay triathlon on Nantucket in June 2001. I had been living a life on Wall Street and wasn't really looking to get married. I had just finished the swimming section of the race and had begun running when I looked over and saw this girl. I ran right over to her, stopped, and stood right next to her while I drank some water. She noticed I was barefoot and asked me how my "tootsies were feeling." Most of the swimmers, including me, had tagged the hand of teammates who were now running on the same sharp rocky road we stood on. I had decided to continue running the rest of race even after tagging my teammate, making me the only barefoot runner . . . still wearing a wetsuit.

During the first thirty seconds of talking with Courtney, I knew she was the one. I must have looked crazy running barefoot with a wetsuit on amidst all the shorts and sneakers, but she never stopped smiling at me. Maybe she thought I was nuts. She understood me, and I was struck by lightning. I never really planned to get married and had never really felt any pressure to settle down. But in an instant, a switch flipped, and I knew I was going to make this woman my wife. It was as simple as that.

On our first date, we went kayaking. I decided to aim for a specific harbor, a distance that wound up taking us eight hours of ocean paddling. We ran out of drinking water four hours into our adventure. I never bring food, so it was pretty epic, especially considering this was her first time paddling. There's nowhere to hide in that tiny kayak, and our date could easily have been a disaster, but the whole time she was chatting and lively and funny as hell. I loved her attitude, and I fell in love with her.

Courtney started traveling with me to races I was participating in, and we had a blast together, no matter the circumstances. In July 2001, I did an adventure race in Scotland, where we camped out in the mountains for several days. The entire time we were attacked by these things called "midgies," little gnats that bite the shit out of your face while you hike or sleep or do anything in that part of the UK. Still, no complaining from Courtney. She always finds the humor and goodness in everything.

From there we flew to visit a friend of mine in Monaco. One evening, we walked past this great, long-established casino, the kind of place where 007 would have gambled. Neither of us really liked to gamble, but on that day we were with friends and feeling frisky, so we decided to make a few life-changing bets on the roulette wheel. We picked numbers: Courtney's was black 8 (her soccer jersey number at Penn State) and I was red 36. If Courtney's number hit, we would immediately leave the casino, fly home to our respective cities, and never speak to each again. If my number hit, we would go straight to the nearest justice of the peace and get married. After all, we each had our passports and a friend to bear witness.

Mind you, we had met for the first time three weeks earlier.

In addition, if the wheel hit on any red number, I would have to get a tattoo, and Courtney could choose its design and location on my body. If it landed on any black number, Courtney would have to get a tattoo and I would pick it out. Well, Courtney wanted a drink before I officially placed the bet, so I sat there waiting for a minute. During the thirty seconds it took her to come back with her drink, right up there on the screen in bright neon letters was red 36. All the blood drained from my face, and I thought she was going to pass out. She kept muttering something about how her older sister would kill her. We nervously laughed it off, and agreed that it didn't count because she wasn't there when it happened. We did play another bet on the roulette wheel — after red 36, what could possibly go wrong? Well, let's just say I have a tattoo to remember it by.

The seed was planted, and my gut feeling was confirmed. When you know what you want, you can make your own luck. Sometimes the universe just shoves you down a path, and you have to be courageous enough to keep going. I knew instantly that I wanted to build a life and family with Courtney. And my instincts proved right. Three months after I met her, I proposed, and she accepted. Ten years and four kids and lots of living later, she's still smiling, although not as much as I am.

You may be thinking, though: what if the wheel had come up black 8? If being a Spartan is about imposing your will, why would you let a casino game dictate the most important decision of your life? Would you have reneged on the deal? Yes, I planned to marry Courtney even if the roulette wheel hit her chosen number. A Spartan never allows chance to interfere with their goals. A Spartan also doesn't mind playing with someone, even a future spouse, to have a memorable experience and gauge her reaction. Think back to the Death Race scenario and how those racers were duped on the last day.

The Rule of Upside Downside holds that before deciding on a course of action, you should think quickly about the positive effects and negative effects of it, weigh them, and decide. I've always been really good at making quick decisions. What's my downside? This is the question I ask myself dozens of times per day. At that Spartan Race at Soldier Hollow, Utah, the sign-up tables had been set up twenty yards beyond an overhead bridge that seemed to me like a better location. Quick upside-downside analysis: What's the upside of moving the tables under the bridge? I'm probably going to get another two hours out of volunteers here because they won't be dying in the sun. What's the downside? While we're moving the sign-up table, twenty-five customers will walk past without giving us their e-mail address. We moved the tables. Think upside-downside at dinner: What's the upside to eating dessert tonight? To having another drink? In the morning, what's the upside or downside to hitting the snooze button? When starting Spartan Race, I decided that the upside — changing thousands of lives — far outweighed the downside, which was that I could lose some money and time. The decision was easy.

I analyze everything based on importance and relevance. That's my nature. A more dramatic example occurred during Hurricane Irene, which hit us pretty hard in Vermont. We were cut off from the rest of the world. A Vermont version of martial law took over in our little town for around ten days. Choppers flew in to bring food and supplies and left with stranded people onboard. We secured diesel from the local fuel supplier, started up all the heavy equipment any farmer or contractor in town had available, and started rebuilding the day after the storm. In many ways it was awesome. Everyone in town took on their respective role based on their expertise, and any animosity disappeared. It was us against mother nature. We were a team with a higher purpose. On a much larger and more profound scale, New York City post-9/11 is arguably the greatest example of this spirit in US history.

When the National Guard and the state authorities arrived, I found myself immediately delegating responsibilities without even realizing it. I was telling people where they should go: "Hey Commander, come here. Commander, you're going to be over here. Who else is in charge? You're in charge? Come here. You're going to take your group. You're over here." In fifteen minutes, I had rerouted everybody from the original plans they had received from their bosses.

"I'm going to need a tractor. Hey you, get a tractor."

"Um, Joe, that's the commander," someone said. "Good! He needs to get a tractor." In retrospect, I was overstepping my bounds, but somehow, in that situation, it worked. After all, we had limited time to open roads and get folks in and out, and the job got done.

Eventually, they gave me a military jacket to wear. Courtney came out in the rain and said, "Of course you're wearing a freaking military jacket now. That's great." It's all part of endurance and quick decision making: being able to put your head down and push ahead while managing people without losing anyone, the way Lewis and Clark did it.

My father was gifted when it came to this kind of thing because he had run construction sites, and I watched him. On a construction job, the financial stakes are high, and everything that can go wrong usually does. If two-by-sixes show up instead of the two-by-fours you actually need, and you're running ten thousand dollars a day in labor — sorry, you just wasted ten thousand dollars. Sound extreme? Look at the "Big Dig" in Boston, a construction project that some estimate went ten billion dollars over budget.

Trading derivatives like I did on Wall Street is similar. One trading mistake can cost you half a million dollars in seconds. You must be able to analyze a given trading situation really fast, make sure you're understanding what's being said, and execute your trade under duress. Every second counts, and every mistake hurts.

Let's say I'm in the middle of a workout. Should I do ten more burpees? The only real downside is an extra sixty seconds of workout time and some additional discomfort. As I've said before, discomfort isn't really a downside if it lowers my expectations and thus my frame of reference for what is normal, good, or ideal. Once that downshift has occurred, I'll have a higher stress tolerance and enjoy the rest of my day more. So if I can spare the sixty seconds, then yes! Ten more burpees! I don't put in the extra work because I love burpees more than everyone else. I do the work because this upside-downside analysis is constantly going through my head. And pretty much every time, the result of the analysis is: Work harder. Be better. Do more.

Upside-downside analysis is useful at any time I need to make a decision. At the restaurant we run in Pittsfield, should I carry the dishes from the table to the sink with two hands or stack everything up and try to carry it in one trip? The downside of two trips is that it takes an extra ten seconds and subjects my legs to more exertion (but not much). The downside of one trip is a much higher risk of breaking stuff, in which case people get upset, we lose money, and we lose a lot of time cleaning up the mess and shopping for new plates. Easy decision.

Should I make this phone call to get more information? Should I send a follow-up e-mail? Should I send a thank-you note? All of these tasks take less time to execute than they do to think about. What's the downside to taking the action?

Sometimes the decision is more complicated but the formula still works. Just the other night my brother-in-law Ian called and invited me to spend some family time in Montauk, New York. Now, I love my family, but travel takes time, and I run a global business. I was in a pickle. Naturally, I turned to my decision-making procedure. Declining the offer and staying in Pittsfield would mean more time to exercise — perhaps a seven-hour bike ride — and manage the business. On the downside, I'd be missing family. Going down to Montauk, though, would involve a twenty-hour bike adventure in the dark — admittedly of my own choosing — plus I'd get to see my family. The risk-reward equation made this a simple decision for me: I biked all the way to Montauk.

Everyone I know thinks that I leap out of bed every morning with an eager smile and a spring in my step. Not a chance. Most of the time I'm pretty unmotivated, but upside-downside analysis is my foolproof method for deciding what to do. I think quickly about potential gains and losses all day every day when making decisions, and then I'm ready to go. Ask yourself: What is the upside versus the downside to sitting on the couch for the next hour? For not taking the elevator and taking the stairs instead? For walking to the store?

At the end of the day, in every one of these decisions, I sacrifice ease and comfort in favor of accomplishments. The downside of my way of life is that it's harder, but I'm okay with that. That's part of being a Spartan. At the end of every day, nothing remains in my body's fuel tank. I fall asleep knowing that I accomplished as much as I possibly could. And when I look back on my life, I want to be able to feel like I did as much as I possibly could have done. That's Spartan pride: looking in the mirror at the end of things, knowing that you did absolutely the best that you could, every single day. It's an amazing feeling, one that everyone should experience.

Spartan Up! Life Lesson No. 3:
Always Remember Those Who Serve

In the days when an ice cream sundae cost much less, a ten-year-old boy entered a hotel coffee shop and sat at a table. A waitress put a glass of water in front of him.

"How much is an ice cream sundae?" the boy asked.

"Fifty cents," replied the waitress. The little boy pulled his hand out of his pocket and studied the coins in his palm. "Well, how much is a plain dish of ice cream?" he inquired.

By now, more people were waiting for a table, and the waitress was growing impatient. "Thirty-five cents," she replied brusquely. The little boy again counted his coins. "I'll have the plain ice cream," he said. The waitress brought the ice cream, put the bill on the table, and walked away. The boy finished the ice cream, paid the cashier, and left. When the waitress came back to wipe down the table, there, placed neatly beside the empty dish, were two nickels and five pennies. You see, he couldn't have the sundae, because he had to have enough left to leave her a tip.

— Author Unknown

8

MAKING YOUR LIMITS VANISH

The only way to find the limits of the possible is by going
beyond them to the impossible.

— SIR ARTHUR C. CLARKE

I N NOVEMBER 2003, five years after my first adventure race, a friend and I were driving from Vermont to see my father in the hospital after he had suffered a heart attack. My friend was behind the wheel, and I was in the passenger seat. At some point, I must have dozed off. When I awoke, I was face-down in frost-covered grass, shivering and disoriented. When I tried to move, I couldn't.

Apparently my buddy had dozed off, too. We veered off the road and drove into a tree. On impact I was ejected from the car. I didn't know it at the time, but my left leg had been torn loose from my hip socket. I was experiencing pain the likes of which I had never felt before, even during the worst moments of my toughest endurance races. This has to be terrible, whatever it is, I thought.

I heard a siren approaching, followed shortly thereafter by the crunch of rapidly nearing footsteps. Someone started speaking, and I remember telling him something along the lines of, no, you can't move me, at least not before you give me some morphine. So they got approval for the morphine, administered it, and then maneuvered me into the ambulance.

I woke up on the emergency room to what sounded like medical professionals discussing my situation. One voice began talking to me. "We have to run you through some tests," it said. "Your leg was ripped out of your hip, and it's behind your body. We need to break your hip and put your leg back where it belongs."

"Do whatever needs to be done," I remember saying.

Time was of the essence, I would find out later. With these injuries, surgeons have six hours to get the leg back in place, or else the internal bleeding would become so severe they would have to amputate the limb.

My leg was saved, but the long-term prognosis for its function wasn't promising, especially considering this new life of endurance racing that I had fallen in love with. In fact, the first five doctors said I would never run again. I didn't know if I could prove the doctors wrong. What I did know was that if the doctors were right, I was fucked. I therefore quickly analyzed the situation and realized I had no choice. I *had* to prove the doctors wrong. If I turned out to be wrong, I'd be no worse off, anyway.

What I needed from the doctors was knowledge. What could I do to increase the chances that I could run again? Could I do any harm? I definitely didn't want to do any more damage. I asked hundreds of questions, reviewed x-rays, and learned everything I could.

After grilling them for days, I formulated my game plan. I bought myself a bunch of Pilates equipment; hired a leading instructor, Christina Gloger; and did Pilates nearly every day for the next six months. Somehow, somewhere, I found the energy to rebuild. It wasn't that I didn't trust the doctors; it was more that I knew I couldn't live with myself if I didn't exhaust all possibilities. You don't get to put another coin in the video game of life. We get one shot at this, and I had to make sure I was doing all I could to recover.

And here I am, still alive and kicking. I've been as good as new ever since. Limits don't vanish magically, and I didn't do anything extraordinary. I simply became informed and then persevered.

My friend, the one who fell asleep at the wheel, suffered a compound fracture in his leg, and he too survived. *We* survived. And knowing that you came so close to death, and cheated it, well, it triggers something inside you. Something I don't think my doctors understood I possessed.

I'm eternally grateful to my doctors for putting me back together, but I'm also glad I didn't listen to their pessimistic long-term prognosis. If I had listened to my doctors then, my life would be entirely different now. I would not be an endurance racer, I would not have started Spartan Race, and I would not be ripping people off their couches to help them shape up. I'm might be sitting on one of those couches myself, in fact, feeling sorry for myself. Instead, I pushed beyond the limits that others wanted to impose.

I see this same spirit of resiliency in our racers all the time. I recently received a note from a young man named Austin who had encountered Spartan Race after trying a mud run put on by another promoter. He had enjoyed the mud run in the same way that he might enjoy a ride at the amusement park or a team-building event at work. It was fun. It whetted his appetite, and he wanted more, so he decided to try a Spartan Race next. He chose the 2012 Pennsylvania Spartan Sprint. He was expecting the same experience he had had at the mud run.

Simply put, we handed him his ass out on the course. "It was the hardest thing I had ever done . . . ever," he wrote to me. "However, I *loved* every second of it, and for the first time in my life, I felt truly alive. The next day, [my friend] and I signed up for the 2012 Tri-State Super, and it once again was the hardest thing I had ever done. The feeling of accomplishment when you cross that finish line is indescribable, but it left a desire for more — much more." The brain rewards hard work.

Two weeks after the Tri-State Super, however, Austin was blindsided when his live-in girlfriend of many years left him without warning. Suddenly, a major part of his life was missing. Like any good Spartan, he responded to the challenge by doing the 2013 Spartan Trifecta, racing the Pennsylvania Sprint, Tri-State Super, and Ottawa Beast.

"Signing up for the races did not fill the void that I was experiencing," he says, "but the physical, mental, and spiritual transformation I experienced along the way certainly did. I've lost close to thirty pounds and my physical condition is better than it's ever been. I'm now obsessed with working out, and I've spent countless hours on spartan.com reading about other people's experiences and transformations. I've accomplished more in 2013 than I ever thought I would. But I still have much more to do."

Feats of Feet and Will

I began running long distances — and then longer and *longer* distances — to push my boundaries and to eliminate my own mental and physical limits, at least as I had perceived them.

At first, I did three-hour races; eventually, I started doing eight-day, self-supported races through remote regions virtually untouched by man. Crazy kinds of races where you could get lost or killed and the jungle would claim your bones. Yet only in pushing myself past these crazy limits did I find true fulfillment and liberation. I found that no amount of career success or money could match the fulfillment I received from competing in and completing these challenges. Maybe I grew addicted to the challenge or the adrenaline, but regardless, I just couldn't resist the drive to push further. Eventually going the distance was no longer the issue; being able to stop was.

When you start an ultraendurance event, the fact that it's going to get ugly at some point is a given. It will reach a dark place where I will think, I can't believe I am putting myself back in this position.

But at some level, that's also the point. Each time I race, I'm testing myself all over again. And as hard as it gets during certain moments in each race, there is also something great about it. The worse the weather, the greater the pain, the more amazing it feels as you take each additional step, pushing through discomfort en route to your destination. If you've never been on a bike seat for fifteen hours straight, you haven't lived! I'm only half-joking. Even during the toughest races, there are so many more miles to go . . . and then, miraculously, it ends. You did it.

It's never easy, but I have learned various mental tricks and techniques to keep me going, to make those limits vanish. Andy talks about this little guy who pops up on your shoulder and gives you every damn good reason to stop. Well, as a distance runner, it's my job to knock him off. Soon enough, he'll be crawling up my leg again, trying to get back onto my shoulder so that he can whisper more negative thoughts into my head. That little guy is nothing if not persistent. So then I need to knock him off me again.

One run where that little guy was especially annoying sticks out in my mind. It was the Ironman Lake Placid, and I was doing it the same week I had already done Badwater and the Vermont 100, which any endurance athlete will tell you is a pretty crazy trifecta of self-inflicted punishment. The run got ugly, so ugly that my legs felt like they were on fire. I needed pain killers but those were off limits for anything other than emergencies, a byproduct of the impact my mom's belief in holistic health had on me. There may come a time when you genuinely need those drugs, like after a bad accident, and if you've used them in lesser situations, they won't work as well when you truly need them to dull intense pain.

On that particular run, the pain and discomfort became so acute that I began to question this whole pursuit of adventure racing. But like all the times before, I focused on putting one foot in front of the other. I convinced myself that time would pass whether

I was moving forward or standing still somewhere, so I would rather be moving forward. I just needed to endure four more hours of hell, knowing that the feeling of accomplishment on the other side of this immediate pain would linger for decades.

During the ninth Eco Challenge in Fiji, and my first, I fully realized that the body can do so much more than we ever thought possible. As insanely hard as that race was, I didn't miss the comforts of back home even during periods of mind-bending exhaustion and deprivation. I wanted food, water, and shelter. That's all I cared about. Period. This more primitive mental state was refreshing, liberating, and empowering. With the artifice of civilization stripped away, I truly felt alive.

I was also struck by how the Fijians we encountered during the race were happy, healthy, strong, self-sufficient, and generous. They lived rich lives without any of the things we are told every day that we need: cars, plastic, toys — none of it. Observing this changed my life.

Every time I run a race, or someone else runs a race, I'm watching a cookie test unfold. To not run, to do something easier instead, is the one-cookie scenario. Running the race, with all the resulting benefits, equals two cookies. It takes discipline to keep running, because every step is another chance to stop and quit. People can say that all you do is put one foot in front of the other, but the reverse holds true as well. You don't even need to set down the weights or hop off a bicycle. All you have to do is *not* take the next step, and you are no longer running. The race is over.

Distance itself becomes an obstacle, and the presence of obstacles makes the races much harder than their mileage would suggest. Even with a race as demanding as an Ironman triathlon, you know what to expect and can train accordingly. There are three obstacles in Ironmans: a swim, and a bike, and a run. So the training can easily be broken down into a series of repetitive motions, all of which need to be done at maximum intensity for a precise distance. You swim in strict form. You bike in strict position. You run on paved roads. Your heart rate stays at one level. It's pure endurance, strength, and yes, speed.

I'm not downplaying the difficulty of the two transitions between these events. I generally spend the last twenty minutes of my swim getting mentally ready for my bike, and I spend the last forty-five minutes on the bike prepping for the run. After swimming an hour, biking feels strange and uncomfortable, and after biking 112 miles, running becomes a whole new experience. But you know when to expect these transition periods, and in your mind, you're ready for them.

In contrast to triathlons, each Spartan Race is unique, dynamic, and unpredictable. The course is integrated into the natural landscape, and every place is different. All elements of the natural terrain are integrated to mess with racers and make them uncomfortable. This unpredictability heightens the demands on the body. Spartan Race fitness involves more than ten thousand variable moves to get through a course.

If you are not fit across every plane of motion, forget about it. Because an obstacle course is unpredictable, our racers have to train for total fitness, addressing each and every component. Full upper-body and core strength must be balanced against running skills. Adaptability, flexibility, and creativity play huge roles in navigating the obstacles. There is no time to get ready for what's next; there is only time to *do* what is next, on the fly. Everything hurts at different times in unpredictable ways, making each obstacle unique even if you've done it before. The rope climb is never just the rope climb — it's the rope climb *after* the countless events you just participated in. The whole race is unpredictable from start to finish, whenever that might be.

This can be maddening for the type A personalities who need

to prepare for and control everything. They can't, just like they can't in life. There are too many variables, too many unknowns, too many twists and turns that cannot be anticipated. In contrast to Ironman, Spartan Race is much more a reflection of life as most of us live it. Discipline is one thing, but another aspect is the complete fluidity. In life, one doesn't know where the start or finish line is. You need a different mindset out on the Spartan course. The rules of the game are constantly shifting, so your frame of reference has to shift along with them.

Spartan Race is also more democratic than organizations like Ironman. An Ironman is 114 miles long, so the kind of person that's probably going to attempt it already has a clearly defined sense of purpose. In contrast, somebody who is struggling and a bit unfocused won't do an Ironman, but they very well could muster the wherewithal to attempt a three-mile Spartan.

In this sense there are great parallels between Spartan Race and the military, which is one reason I named this obstacle-racing enterprise after a legendary military force from ancient times. Very little goes exactly as planned in battle, and to use a sports metaphor, the history of war is filled with tremendous upset victories. So if you took that exacting Ironman mentality and training into the theater of war, you might very well get crushed by some unforeseen turn of events. You need to rewire your brain to constantly shift its frame of reference as circumstances change. That's how you survive in battle and succeed in life.

Expectations, when they're not met, lead to frustration. If you're expecting a three-mile run, and it ends up being five miles, you're frustrated and upset. In the Spartan Race, we make the unexpected fun. If you have no expectations, you are less likely to be upset when you are confronted with obstacles that catch you off guard.

Sharpening Your Focus

I also started running long distances to strip a lot of the clutter from my mind. Distance events force you to focus. In contrast, our society likes to stay distracted, always chasing the next shiny object. We train to keep our minds busy, and they become willing accomplices. Soon we have no choice: we are slaves to our anxious, darting minds and the constant stream of useless mental chitchat. This sort of mental chatter isn't really thinking; it's just neurological white noise, a distraction from what really matters.

I benefit particularly from this sort of focus because I have a severe case of ADD. We used to be hunter-gatherers, and when we became an agrarian society, those hunter-gatherer genes remained in the population. I and other ADD sufferers like me inherited at least some of them. A hunter-gatherer was either hunting or being hunted, so he or she was constantly monitoring the environment, like an air-traffic controller analyzing moving blips.

The stillness of mind we achieve in endurance racing isn't always easy to replicate, but it's important to heighten your focus in everyday life. Doing so requires fencing off your brain from all the clutter that invades it all day through phones and computers. For starters, sleep is everything when it comes to achieving mental focus and physical preparedness. In fact, living with the mindset "I'll sleep when I'm dead" may get you there quite a bit faster!

A healthy lifestyle includes at least seven hours of uninterrupted sleep per night. Without it, you're more likely to suffer from obesity, cognitive decline, type 2 diabetes, heart disease, and perhaps even cancer. One reason may be that sleep deprivation decreases insulin sensitivity. What that means is that your cells don't recognize the hormone whose job it is to usher glucose (blood sugar) into cells.

Left stranded in your bloodstream, that excess glucose tends to lead to weight gain.

To sleep longer and more soundly, avoid consuming caffeine after 3:00 P.M. Caffeine is a stimulant that stays in your system for more than six hours! Even if you don't feel jittery, caffeine is still pinging your sympathetic nervous system. You should also avoid using laptops, iPads, and cell phones for at least an hour or two before bedtime. The intense blue light emitted by many of today's most popular gadgets shine directly into the eyeballs, confusing the brain, suppressing melatonin production, and disrupting the circadian rhythm developed over hundreds of thousands of years, whereby we sleep and awaken by the rising and falling of the sun.

Exercise and a healthy diet promote restful sleep. If you work out hard, you sleep well. If you eat well, you sleep well. Our body needs to work each and every day, and typing all day on the computer doesn't count. You have to sweat and your heart has to pump. If you do that, you're likely to sleep well. You don't need sleep-enhancing pills or a study from a medical journal to confirm this. Just try it. But when that alarm goes off in the morning, don't hit snooze!

Total mind-body-spirit fitness is the Spartan ideal. History's elite warriors have known that to win on the real battlefield, you must first win on the battlefield of your mind. This requires mastering your emotions and allowing your intellect to decide what's important. You must be able to prioritize. How can you achieve greatness if you are constantly sidetracked by trivial pursuits? You must develop a mind strong enough to resist distractions and temptations. Greatness doesn't come from obsessing over the trivial events of the day and checking your social media accounts twenty times an hour.

If we turn the clock back, we will actually perform better in life. It's completely contrary to everything we've been told. This march toward modernization and convenience has taken us in the wrong direction. The Spartan Race is a reaction against all of that. The Spartan Race is an attempt to stem the tide, to get back to the basics of human nature and mechanics — and good health.

The question may arise in your mind: Why must I actually *do* a Spartan Race? Can't I just take lessons like working out, eating better, and sleeping well and apply them to my life? Can I just read this book? You could, but it wouldn't be the same. A Spartan proves himself or herself through actions, not words. And Spartans know that the race itself is a more formidable opponent than the other competitors. In fact, you have a bond with your competitors because you share the crucible experience and the goal of surviving whatever is thrown at you. Sometimes in life, you just have to dive in, and such is the case with a Spartan Race. The ice water hitting your body will make you feel alive and compel you to new heights out on the course.

I believe we all need to be tested; otherwise, how do we discover what we're made of? Signing up for a competitive event commits you to crushing your known limits. You crush it when you find yourself in the zone, when it all falls together and nothing that crops up can get to you. Unpredictability no longer matters, because you innately have the answers, and you are physically prepared for the challenge.

Without that self-imposed pressure, it can be hard for people to stay on track. The event holds you accountable to meeting your goals. When you run a Spartan Race, you are saying that you have the courage to change your lifestyle, to leave behind your deeply ingrained patterns, to become a different and better person. Not just to fly but to soar.

The rewards are substantial. "If it weren't for this Spartan event, I might have always thought the big guys were stronger than me," wrote Spartan competitor Vanessa Runs in a blog post. "Above all, I learned to not be intimidated. To be confident in my fitness. And that in the end, maybe the life awards don't go to the biggest guys. Maybe it's better to be tiny. To slip easily under every obstacle."

Whether or not you run an obstacle race, the bigger question is preparing for a richer and fuller life. The principles underpinning the Spartan way can help you succeed at anything. The first key to the Spartan lifestyle is keeping to the big picture. It's not healthy to get too focused on any one aspect of your life. If you do, it will almost inevitably be to the detriment of others. Healthy foods, healthy attitude, healthy relationships, healthy mind, and healthy body together define a complete Spartan lifestyle — the Spartan code in action.

Why do I "go the distance"? And is all that effort worth it in the end? For the answer, I need look back no further than to my father and his failing heart, the combination that set the stage for my terrible car accident when I went to visit him in 2003. In 2013, I arrived at Saint Francis Hospital in Long Island to find my dad unconscious and on life support. His feet had turned black from poor circulation, the catheters sticking out of him made him look like a voodoo doll, and a ventilator was helping him to breathe when every breath could well be his last. My dad had never paid much attention to his health. He didn't exercise, and he hated fruits and vegetables. Mostly his diet consisted of manufactured and highly processed foods, which explains his heart disease and diabetes.

Over the past decade, he had suffered five heart attacks, received a handful of stents, and had several blood transfusions, for starters. He had been dead, technically, for six minutes the day before, but somehow he had pulled out of it again.

As much as I loved my dad, I couldn't just sit there all morning looking at him lifeless on that table. So I left the hospital for a while and found a gym down the street called the Fitness Loft. I asked the receptionist if I could get a workout in. "You have to be a member," she said. I noticed a flyer for Spartan Race on the counter, and told the girl I was one of the event's founders. She smiled and said, "In that case, come on in. We think what you guys do is so badass."

At some point during the next ninety minutes, while I was torturing myself in the gym, I stopped for a moment and realized how privileged I was. My poor dad's health had turned him into a shadow of a human being, let alone his once-imposing self. At this point, it was impossible for him to push his body in the gym and reclaim his health. I realized at that moment how precious health really is. How could I not work out? I thought. How could anyone not work out?

When I tell people to get off the damn couch and eat real food, they sometimes assume I'm running from death, and they play the carpe diem card: "Why toil for your health when you could just get hit by a car tomorrow? Enjoy your life while you can, and do everything in moderation." Really? Well, what about when you're in a hospital bed on a respirator and taking twenty-six different medications like my dad was in the hospital next door — try to enjoy life then! At Spartan Race, it's not that we're trying to avoid death; we're trying to enjoy our lives fully, to wring every wonderful drop out of life that we possibly can.

The use of our body is a privilege, one that millions of people forget, neglect, and forfeit. Too many forget what enjoying life really means. And before they know it, carpe diem, Latin for "seize the day," turns into mea culpa. Latin for "my bad."

I was lucky enough to have been wired from an early age to live a healthy life. My hope is that Spartan parents will teach their kids to live in a way that will keep them out of the emergency room later in life. That they'll give them the knowledge of health and fitness and physical activity and help them to enjoy a healthy, long, and happy life.

A healthy life is a life without limits.

In the classic novel *The Lord of the Rings*, the young Hobbit Frodo must say goodbye to his loved ones and proceed on his quest to destroy the One Ring of Power on his own as war looms on the horizon.

He tells his friend, the noble wizard Gandalf, "I wish none of this had happened."

Gandalf's reply is one of the greatest in all of literature. He says, "So do all who live to see such times. But that is not for them to decide. All we have to decide is what to do with the time that is given to us . . ."

To me, Gandalf is saying that we live in a world of pain and conflict, and that death is inevitable for all of us. But we do have one great source of power, and that is the fact that we can decide what to do with the time we have on earth, and that the best of those decisions are the ones that make the world a better place. That's what the Spartans did. In a small way, that is what I'm trying to do with Spartan Race.

9

TRANSFORMANCE: FORGING NEW BONDS

A child without discipline is a child without love.

— MR. ROGERS

MY WIFE COURTNEY grew up in the "perfect" American family, almost like something out of *Leave It to Beaver* or *Father Knows Best*. They would hold hands at the dinner table and pray before eating. I wasn't sure those kinds of things actually happened outside of old black-and-white television shows, but I saw it with my own eyes after meeting Courtney's family.

She's Irish, and all the men in her family were in law enforcement. They all worked hard and played hard, too. Each family member, male and female, pursued at least one sport with hard-charging intensity, which helped him or her grow as individuals while binding them as a unit. Courtney was great at soccer and eventually became the captain of her team in college, taking them to the "final four" during her senior year. Aside from her competitive fire on the soccer field, she is pretty laid back and easygoing otherwise . . . as anyone dealing with me would have to be.

Courtney and I have four children. As of this writing, Jack is seven years old, Charlie is five, Catherine is four, and Alexandra is nine months. We knew we wanted a big family and thought carefully about planning and creating it. Now that we are surrounded by children, we approach parenting with a plan and goals. For example, we wanted to teach our children languages besides English from an early age, when their brains were most receptive to learning them. Jack and Charlie both are learning Mandarin. What's more, Charlie, our five-year-old son, has swum a mile (wearing a life jacket, of course). They all do two hours a day of kung fu, and Jack skis fifty-plus days a year. Catherine has done sets of three hundred burpees. We have been trying to get Alexandra to do burpees, but at this point the best we can get is burps.

Courtney and I are very concerned that one of our children could be "pushed over the edge" and to a place where they no longer like an activity — in which case our strategy would have backfired. Rather than mastering an activity, they would lose interest in it.

When we're wading through, say, a difficult swim, I simply ask, "Do you want to stop?" I always tell them they can achieve their goal another time. They're smart kids, and the more they know about an activity's difficulty, the prouder they become about succeeding at it. With language, our policy is simple: you can watch as much television as you want as long as it is in Mandarin.

Our theory is the children inherently want to push themselves, that this is their natural state of affairs. If you send kids out for recess, what happens? They climb and swing and tumble for the sheer joy of their own movement. Think back to when you were a kid. I'll bet that when you came upon a puddle, you didn't walk around it; you gleefully splashed right through it. Kids who aren't yet brainwashed by electronic media go outside to play, explore, and get dirty. They squat down to dig in the sand with impeccable flexibility and balance.

Kids push themselves mentally, too, if we let them. Unfortunately, we push them in the other direction. They gravitate to the couch at an age when they should be drawn instead to fresh air and sunshine.

In this age of video games and smartphones and iPads, too often we are tempted to give our children a screen, the twenty-first century's answer to babysitting, yet by doing so we are further dulling their natural impulse to be active beings. The decline of physical activity among children and young people is a worldwide phenomenon. A recent study by New Zealand researchers found that between the ages of three and five, physical activity declines by roughly half, a decrease that's maintained through age seven, which was the endpoint for the study. Another recent study in Britain found that physical activity decreases among British youths during early adolescence. So during the years when lifelong habits are formed, kids today become more sedentary and less active, which harms everything from their health to their self-esteem.

This isn't a natural state of affairs, either. Nested within each of our bodies and minds, from the moment of birth until the moment of death, is an inborn impulse to grow, heal, build mastery, fulfill our potential, and naturally correct our own course when we drift or are knocked off it. This trait is called *transformance,* and anyone who has ever watched a two-year-old trying to master walking up and down stairs has witnessed this trait in action. The toddler will determinedly make his way up and down, not because anyone told him to or because he is trying to "get in shape," as any number of grown-ups do on StairMasters at the gym.

In fact, a two-year-old isn't even capable of conscious intention at this stage of development. He or she may fall and cry, but soon they're at it again, a look of pride spreading on their face with every small victory. A child will reject someone's hand unless they're too unsteady for the next step, in which case they'll grasp it in order to continue. This desire to master a task, even in the face of challenges and hard work, is incredible to watch.

Think also of older children on a playground. They're running, jumping, laughing, and having a ball. They're on the monkey bars, the ladders, pumping on the swing, jumping from death-defying heights, walking the balance beam, persisting until they master each feat in turn. The only reward is the joy that comes from accomplishing something new. They revel in what their bodies can do and naturally push the limits until they conquer the next new obstacle. Falls, bruises, scrapes — if not serious — become badges of courage, marks of how hard they are playing and how far they are pushing themselves.

When we are kids, we want to be popular, good at sports, make good grades, receive parental approval. But we don't necessarily know how to achieve that. The answer to all of these desires generally comes down to *work harder*. Practice more hours, study more hours, put more effort into changing your habits.

Nearly everyone I have ever known has the desire to improve their life in some way. So if they want to improve their lives, why don't they? I've trained hundreds of people who all say some variation on the following:

"I want to get into better shape."

"I want to lose twenty pounds."

These people tell me stories about how they have tried this exercise program or that diet and about how it didn't work. So why have so many of these individuals failed to achieve their goals?

It's not normal in our society to go out for a run on a Sunday morning and push yourself to the point where the pain is etched into your face. Similarly, it's not normal for a business executive to wake up every morning and knock out one hundred burpees. It's not normal, that is, unless you are getting in shape for a special event, or unless you are training for some specific goal.

This is why I always tell people: "Just sign up. Don't worry about whether you are in good enough shape — just sign up." When people sign up for a Spartan Race, they start training harder. They are motivated to complete the course, so they start pushing themselves to exhaustion during their daily workouts. It's normal to train really hard before an event, so they do. And when they get to the event, they are in the kind of shape that they had hoped they would be, and they are able to cross the finish line along with everyone else.

I can't count the number of people we have convinced to sign up for a race who then got hooked and transformed. A friend — let's call her Sabrina — who was recently divorced had gained some weight, and she was in the beginning of a mild depression. It took a while to convince her to sign up, but by getting her friends involved, she finally took the bait. Once Sabrina signed up the magic happened: daily training, new friends, commitment, a new purpose, and so forth.

To understand why some people succeed and why some people don't, you have to look at their assumptions of what is normal. These assumptions will drive their motivation. To achieve more, people must change their outlook. They must change their frame of reference.

Think of the teenager who wants to get better grades. At night, he thinks it's normal to do homework for one hour and play video games for two hours. What would happen if suddenly he thought it was normal to study four hours a night?

The kid who wants to make the basketball team — he thought it was normal to practice for one hour per day after school, including one hundred practice free throws. What would happen if suddenly he thought it was normal to practice for three hours per day and to shoot five hundred practice free throws?

Admittedly, our kids will have a lot of built-in advantages that other, equally remarkable children don't. Take Matthias Vescelus. He has been a fighter all his life. When he was three months old, he lost both eyes to bilateral retinoblastoma, a rare cancerous tumor. When he was three years old, one of his siblings finished a Spartan Race. Matthias was determined to complete one, too. It took him a year of preparation, but at age four, he completed a Spartan Race for kids in Indiana. It was an epic event for the entire family, bringing everyone closer together.

There are phases you'll go through when experiencing transformance, and you can use them to add momentum to your progress.

Phase 1) When you're transforming, you will enter a dark phase where you feel like you are against the wall or afraid. That's why so many people seek out ultraendurance events and obstacles — there's an attraction to this dark phase even though it's so hard to break through.

If you just can't get over an obstacle, if you're stuck, having serious issues, afraid, exhausted, you've hit a dark phase. This happens when we take folks out into the woods where there's no trail. For many people, it's scary at first but then becomes liberating.

Phase 2) The second phase involves getting comfortable. It's easier to emerge from the dark phase and become more comfortable if others are around you and working toward the same goal. That is why Spartan Race is so powerful: You are with ten thousand others doing the same thing and breaking out of that dark, uncomfortable, tired place and overcoming obstacles.

Phase 3) The third phase is mastery. You conquered a challenge, or at least see that it's possible to do so, and then you can't get enough of it.

Take One for the Team

The fighting spirit needs to be rekindled in us all. Spartan Race is an example of a place where this can happen. However, places and events that spark team spirit are even more important! Spartan Race teams join up together, encourage one another, jockey for position, then save each other's asses when the chips are down. That's one of the most awesome aspects of the race. The camaraderie among

Spartan racers is unlike anything you'll see in the endurance world, pro sports, or corporate America. Perhaps only the military offers a parallel.

Fifty-five-year-old Cathy Bergman and her friends offer living proof of this team mentality. In the fall of 2011, a friend of Cathy's ran a Spartan Sprint in New York and sent Cathy photos of the experience. "Although crawling through mud under barbed wire is not generally a favorite pastime of most women in their middle fifties, to me it looked like great fun," Cathy recalls.

When she visited the Spartan Race website, she noticed that a Spartan Sprint was schedule for June 2012 in Mont Tremblant, Quebec, a mere fifteen minutes from her front door. She decided to go for it, but even with a year to prepare, this was a tall order. She was so out of shape and had been that way for so long that it was hard for her to stand up without assistance, let alone run an obstacle race on her own. Yet she found a personal trainer willing to help her and committed herself to eating clean. What's more, she recruited thirteen friends and neighbors to form a team for the race. These ladies called themselves the Domaine Alarie Spartans.

The section of her property that in years past had been the site of family picnics and barbecues was converted into a Spartan training ground. A few dozen middle-aged women began training like they were in Special Ops. Cathy describes what happened next: "Weekend after weekend, friends and neighbors crawled on their stomachs under netting, pulled tires through the sand, lifted weights, chucked spears, did endless pushups and pull-ups and ran from one end of the beach to the other, working on cardio and endurance in anticipation of the upcoming race."

At the starting line of the race, Cathy weighed 125 pounds, 170 pounds less than when she started. In other words, she had already won before the race began. At the end of the race, "We were muddy, bloody, and soaked to the skin, but nothing dampened the exhilaration of our journey to Sparta," says Cathy. "Having been to Sparta and left with a smile, we learned that it was not the finish line that counted, it was what it took to get to the finish line and the wonderful friendships that were forged along the way."

In reality, everyone wants to be successful, as Cathy and her teammates ultimately were. But so many people just don't know how to begin. Spartan racing is a playground for adults, one that can awaken this primal force of transformance within all of us. Too often, the transformance pulse within adults grows fainter from exhaustion, poor diet, trauma, defeat, criticism, helplessness, and routines that are deadening instead of vitalizing.

Several features of Spartan racing awaken transformation:

1. Reconnecting with our bodies, a side effect of which can be the reawakening of sexual response.
2. Achievement of mastery, which builds confidence, grace, and focus.
3. Connection to others, because well-being, serenity, and mastery make it easier to love, easier to support our family, friends, and community, and easier to make the world a better place.

I can't overstress the importance of mastery. You may remember rope climbs from PE class in elementary school. Maybe you haven't done once since. They're not easy, in part because your body is a much heavier load than it was in grade school. By the time you reach this obstacle on a Spartan course, chances are you're already pretty beat up from fatigue and mud and other elements. The rope extends above a water-filled pit, so the first imperative, especially on cold days, is to keep your hands dry; otherwise, they might cramp as you grasp the rope, which is an inch thick. Regardless, you have to reach as high as you can, grasp the rope, and then clench your core to pull up your knees. The upward climb is a great test of strength. If any muscle gives way before you reach the top and ring the bell, signifying success, a hard fall will end with a splash into the mud pit below. Rather than offering a helping hand, we issue a penalty: thirty more burpees.

Pulling your own weight above earth and defying gravity while dangling from a thick rope is extremely liberating. Mastering an obstacle like the rope climb leads to the robust self-confidence to face the next challenge, along with positive emotions such as pride and self-appreciation. Such positive emotions nourish healthy self-esteem and well-being without tipping over into arrogance. Everybody finds something in a Spartan Race that they can't do well. Not yet, anyway.

The rope climb is the obstacle that gives me the most trouble. From an early age, I had trouble with pull-ups or even just getting my body up and over fences. Most people who master the rope climb use their feet as a clamp to lock themselves in place while they reach up to inch higher. I've never quite mastered the foot lock, and I always rely too heavily on my upper body to work my way up. As with anything else, though, I keep practicing in an attempt to master it. I like to focus on the things in life that I don't do well, my weaknesses and shortcomings, so the rope climb has become part of my daily routine.

Finally, Spartan racing nurtures and embodies a sense of community ("Yes, you can do it!") that will offer support to those who find their limits. At an eight-foot wall, twelve miles into a Beast Race, you will find people boosting, hoisting, and assisting others over, and then receiving assistance in turn. We find the courage to go to the edge of our capacities only when we no longer fear encountering our limits. For this, we need to trust that there will be assistance when we need it, so we don't languish in shame or defeat. These elements allow individuals who commit to a Spartan Race to experience some form of empowerment and victory that fuels more energy, determination, and joyful exploration. And they allow them to *share* it. It is infectious.

When Spartans gather at the starting line, they are no longer competitors. They are no longer strangers. They are Spartans. They become part of a new family, a new team, all of whose members strive to be better in mind, body, and spirit. Look around and you see different skin colors, different ages, different clothing styles, and different body shapes reflecting different fitness levels. And when the race starts, they're all in it together. When you run a marathon or a 10K, you may run with friends, but you don't "help" each other. In Spartan Races, you can actually help friends, teammates, or complete strangers overcome obstacles. Spartans help each other, and no Spartan gets left behind.

If Spartan Races seem difficult to someone without physical limitations, they must seem impossible for someone in a wheel-chair. The rugged terrain would seem hard to navigate, the mud impenetrable. And how the hell would you climb over a greased wall or get underneath barbed wire? Without a team to assist, it would seem impossible.

Michael Mills is a T-12 paraplegic, the victim of a head-on collision with a drunk driver in 1993. In an instant, his entire universe changed. He retained control of his hands and arms, as well as his trunk, but lost most of the use of his legs and hip flexors. Nobody would have blamed him if he withdrew from life to live out his remaining days in solitude, bitter over the hand he had been dealt. Instead, he's been tackling wheelchair racing since 1996, competing in more than 160 road-and-track races, even representing the United States in international events.

Mills decided in August 2012 to sign up to compete in a Spartan Race scheduled for Conyers, Georgia, on March 9, 2013. It wasn't a decision he made or a commitment he entered into casually, either. "I remember being scared to hit the payment button," he recalls. "I knew when I did that there would be no turning back. The thought of doing something I had never done before terrified me, but at the same time I was excited to embark on a new adventure for disabled sports."

Mind you, endurance events aren't Mills' sole preoccupation or calling in life. He works an eight-hour day to support his wife and family, so he needs to squeeze in his workouts before and after work while still leaving time to parent and be a good husband. Somehow, though, he managed. "Once I started training for the Spartan Race, I found something deep inside of me that I really didn't know I had," he says. "It's an even stronger willpower and determination."

As part of his prep, Mills became the first paralyzed person to climb Stone Mountain in Georgia, summiting the mountain along with a team of fellow Spartans. The climb took four hours since Mills was crawling on his hands and knees. This isn't about going it alone; it's about becoming part of something bigger than yourself. Spartans leave no one behind. It is great to push yourself alone, but it is even greater to compete along with friends and acquaintances to reach a new level.

When you race as a team there is a new psychological factor to consider. There will be moments when your team members are stronger or weaker than you. These dynamics will test your ability to remain rational and supportive and to keep your focus on the benefit of the team. Total dedication to your team is every bit as important in life as it is on the course.

"When I see something that looks difficult, it makes me want to do it," Mills told me. "My fear left me, my anxiety turned to excitement, and I knew that this was the year for me to do amazing things."

Family Matters

With our emphasis on personal responsibility and teamwork, it may come as no surprise that Spartan Race emphasizes parenting and family. A family that lives the Spartan code stays together. Bonds are strengthened after they're stretched. That is why we host events that are family oriented and have a place for men, women, and children to share a healthy experience of overcoming obstacles together. We want families to take home the experience and then live it moving forward.

In case you're wondering, my kids have all run at least junior versions of Spartan Races. And so have Andy's. I want them to enjoy all those intellectual and physical advantages later in life. Kids on their own are not going to all of a sudden say, "You know what? We've got to go out and hunt and trap animals. We have to go work out for two hours instead of playing online games." The key is to motivate them without burning them out, without causing them to go in the other direction in reaction to such discipline. If you push too hard, they rebel and do the opposite. This challenge is the most delicate line to balance. Too far one way or the other makes your children and the world a different place.

When we parent correctly, we end up with children like Ella Kociuba. At the age of thirteen, she suffered a horseback riding accident that left her spine fractured. With a surgery that revealed a more serious problem, doctors were promising she would be "normal," but sports and competition were out of the question. But the competitive young lady in her would hear nothing of it. Rather than downshift her physical activity due to her injuries, she decided to give the Spartan Race a try. This has transformed her mentally, emotionally, and physically. She became the athlete she never was growing up. She finally made newspapers and became the champion she always dreamed of being.

Parents shape their children, and parenting has changed me in many ways, too. With these endurance races, no matter who you are, this little voice bends your ear. With me, now, it's not just "You can't do this; just give up; stop and go grab a beer." Now that little person starts saying, "Gee, what are you doing out here for four hours? Why aren't you at home with your kids?" That's a tough argument to counter. When you have kids, to not be with them . . . well, that's an argument I lose every time.

Everyone with kids has to work and figure out how to balance, but at the end of the day, you can't get that time back with your kids. I'm a big believer in talking to old-timers and getting as much knowledge as I can from those who have already lived. My friend Al, who is past seventy now, has helped guide me through the last twenty years of my life. He always seems to have it right, like many old-timers do. He said early on, "Do not miss time with your kids. You will regret it, and you don't get a do over." Just ask anyone with older children — they all say, "Spend time with your kids. It goes really fast."

Like everyone else, though, I have to adapt to the myriad demands of my life — my family, my business, my marriage — and also still carve out time for my own health, as I always have. As I always will. The frame of reference is just different. And I'm a Spartan. I adapt.

Communication has always been central to the Spartan way. Racing as a team requires clear and concise communication. Can you imagine climbing Mount Everest with a team and not communicating well? By openly communicating, we ensure that we are accurately informed and aware of what other team members are going through. In Spartan Races, we are pushing our limits, and when doing so, communicating with others becomes even more critical.

You can't parent—you can't lead, period—if you don't communicate. So we came up with what we call the "Spartan Up! Communication Principles":

- Actively listen. Most people would benefit from speaking less and listening more. You can always learn from other people's experiences, but first you have to hear them. Listening is a sign of respect, and it shows that you value what the other person has to say. Some would argue that this is the reason we have two ears and one mouth.

- Add value. In any situation, we can enhance or detract from the experience of those around us. We can help to clear the dishes, keep an eye on the kids, smile and bring positive energy to the room. People will invite you back if they enjoyed their own experience more as a result of our presence.

- Don't complain. Nothing productive comes from the statement "This sucks." When we complain, we are implicitly shifting responsibility for our situation onto someone else and blaming them for our unhappiness. If the situation could be better, we can take responsibility for it and volunteer to provide solutions to improve our lot.

- Inform but don't dictate. We know what's best for us, but we can never truly know what's best for another person. Life is complicated, and often it's hard to know the best course of action. Share information freely, but allow people to decide their own fate. Allow them to take responsibility for their own happiness.

- Bring out the best in others. We can encourage people to be the best person they can be by giving them credit for what they're good at, by telling them how they have inspired us, by explaining to them how our lives are better because of them. By being supportive, we can help others to build self-confidence, to achieve more in life, to fully realize their potential. Living a Spartan life means expressing the full potential of your entire person.
- Be open and receptive. Seeing the world from someone else's perspective can shift our beliefs, and that's a good thing. To expand our own horizons, we need to be willing to try new things and explore new beliefs.
- Smile. Be happy. By smiling, we remind others, "It's not so bad, everything will be okay." By exuding happiness, we are saying: "We are grateful to be where we are and with the people around us."

I attend as many Spartan Races as I possibly can, and I greet as many racers as I possibly can, looking them in the eye and urging them on. It's my way of connecting with them, and it means a lot, or so I've been told. I feel like I get more out of these interactions than the racers do, though.

Researchers have explored the benefits of gratitude practice in daily life and in the face of hardship. Building a good gratitude practice can help us face and overcome challenges and can be an essential part of the mental preparation for an endurance race. Even in the hardest moments, finding something to be grateful for (i.e., the burning in my legs means that I am strong enough to work this hard; at least I'm not carrying a sixty-pound cement bag anymore) can carry us through, bolster endurance, flood the brain with all the neurochemicals related to positive emotions.

Bob Emmons, a professor of psychology at the University of California–Davis, has researched gratitude as a concept. He has found that people who have a daily gratitude practice also:

- Consistently experience more positive emotions
- Feel more alert, energetic, enthused, alive
- Sleep better
- Have lower blood pressure
- Are more likely to accomplish personal goals
- Are more likely to exercise and stick with a self-improvement program like losing weight

We are a culture that has become shortsighted. Spearmint gum has a nice, perky flavor (for about three minutes), but eating it over and over again dulls your taste buds so they can't pick up on the subtle flavors of fine wine. I have to give a hand to the team that set up Cassini-Huygens, an unmanned spacecraft sent to Mars; they really show what it means to master the cookie test. Imagine if every word you spoke took an hour to get into the ear of the person you were talking to, and then it took another hour for them to nod their head and acknowledge that they heard what you said. That was pretty much the situation between these guys and the spacecraft; and if anything is patience, *that* is. They started building the craft in 1977 and launched it in 1997, and the primary mission was completed in 2008. Lots of waiting, but a huge payoff.

This isn't just an individual problem; it's a global problem with enormous implications for humanity and the fate of our planet. On a macro level, various examples of "taking the cookie now" have led to regional, national, and global disasters. Consider the plastic bag epidemic worldwide, or the Great Pacific Garbage Patch, a floating mass of plastic waste the size of California. People and corporations all over the world "take the cookie now" by using and discarding plastic bags, packaging, and single-use products, polluting the environment as a consequence.

Conversely, many American Indian tribes believe in purposely limiting their population growth in order not to overburden their ecosystem. The "taking the cookie now" choice would be to multiply and consume as much as desired now and deal with the consequences later.

Less is more. Specifically, less "stuff" is more. Stuff owns you, you don't own it. Just look at Spartan Race, Inc. It's a good business. It's exciting, it's staffed by awesome Spartans, and it's incredibly gratifying that we are changing lives. But it is also twenty-hour days, with hundreds of e-mails and phone calls. Is that any way to live? If you believe the American dream, owning a big house is the way to happiness. Really? Taxes, mowing, maintenance, cleaning, repairs . . . Believe me, it doesn't create happiness, it just makes you work more to pay the bills. Besides, everything that you see as "wrong" with the house or the things in it weighs on you. Think about how free you feel on vacation — why? Because you don't own the hotel room or the car you rented, and you're not sweating all the other things you own back home. Are they locked up? Broken? Do they need to be cleaned?

We are on the planet for a very short time, and that is our most precious asset: our time. In light of that fact, we need to maximize our time here, not by worrying about all the stuff we have accumulated but by staying healthy and doing great things every day. We also want to be good stewards of our planet. These two things — child rearing and environmental protection — are intimately connected in our mind. We want to raise good kids who will grow up respecting and preserving the natural world, but we also think it's our responsibility to hand them a world that we have taken care of to the best of our ability.

So what are the great things to do every day? Invest in the people around you. Spartan relationships are strong. Build them strong and keep them that way. Invest in developing self-awareness and self-mastery. Take advantage of opportunities to learn all the time. Discover the causes that you really care about and find ways to support them. Act on your conscience. Lead by your actions and your character. A true Spartan life starts with total physical fitness, but it encompasses emotional and intellectual fitness as well.

The Spartan life is as simple — and as hard — as applying your common sense. Throw the norm out the window. For most people in our contemporary Western culture, "normal" is whatever is easy or provides instant gratification. Fast food is normal, consuming alcohol is normal, not exercising is normal, cutting corners is normal, watching hours of TV every day is normal, cheating is normal . . . Common sense tells you that this definition of normal is unhealthy, unsatisfying, and degrading. So fuck normal and follow your common sense. Exercise your body, heart, and mind.

Spartan Up! Life Lesson No. 4: Giving When It Counts, No Matter the Cost

Many years ago, when a friend worked as a volunteer at a hospital, I got to know a little girl named Liz who was suffering from a rare disease that threatened her life. Her only chance of recovery appeared to be a blood transfusion from her five-year-old brother, who had miraculously survived the same disease and had developed the antibodies needed to combat it.

The doctor explained the situation to her little brother and asked the boy if he would be willing to give his blood to his sister. My friend saw him hesitate for only a moment before taking a deep breath and saying, "Yes, I'll do it if it will save her." As the transfusion progressed, he lay in bed next to his sister and smiled, as we all did, seeing the color returning to her cheek. Then his face grew pale and his smile faded. He looked up at the doctor and asked with a trembling voice, "Will I start to die right away?" Being young, the little boy had misunderstood the doctor; he thought he was going to have to give his sister all of his blood in order to save her.

10

THE FINISH LINE: BECOMING SPARTAN

Whether you think you can, or you think you can't — you are right.

— HENRY FORD

I MEET SPARTANS ALMOST every day. Some of them are part of our organization. Far more of them participate in our races. And then there are others who are Spartans in spirit and deed.

Sir Richard Branson, the multibillionaire founder of the Virgin Group, is, in many ways, a quintessential Spartan. Virgin comprises more than four hundred companies, and Branson himself is a natural-born adventurer. He owns an airline, of course, and he's even launched a space tourism company called Virgin Galactic. So he knows a thing or two about traveling long distances through unfamiliar terrain.

In late 2013, I spent a weekend in the British Virgin Islands with him and a small group of people. On our last day there, Branson announced that he wanted to go sailing. The weather was lousy and deteriorating by the moment, and word was that the sea was wild and choppy. I heard several people, including a few who were experienced sailors, explaining to Branson why taking out his catamaran was a bad idea and perhaps even dangerous.

He was undaunted. "Who wants to go?" he asked.

No one else wanted to go. But I told him, "If you're going, I'm going."

So he, two buddies of his, and I boarded his eighteen-foot Hobie catamaran and headed out into the bay. The winds were gusting so hard that we were *flying* in no time. The water was choppy as hell, and we were getting buckets of water tossed in our face. Sometimes the whole boat would practically be underwater, but Branson was undaunted. His zest for life was on full display, and he was clearly in his element, even if the rest of us were out of ours and drenched.

We navigated our way to an island Branson owns called Mosquito. As we were walking around the island, a group of guys — employees of his, I assume — insisted, "Hey, we'll take you back." Well, a few minutes later, I looked over and there was Branson, at sixty-three years old, wrestling with this heavy boat and getting it back in the water all by himself. Mind you, this boat was probably twenty times heavier than the one the Olympic wrestling coach couldn't handle in one of the earlier anecdotes of the book.

This is a microcosm of why Branson is as successful as he is and why he's achieved all that he has. He's always happy, and his frame of reference is always in place, so he never loses perspective on what matters and what doesn't. You would think he'd be surrounded by opulence and be over the top, but that's not him. He's working hard every day, breathing heavy and sweating, doing all those things that I've mentioned in this book.

When we were walking around the island, I finally just had to stop and ask: "Sir Richard, Spartan Race is growing by leaps and bounds, and I'm trying to manage it all, but you've got four hundred companies! How do you do it?"

"The key is delegation," he said.

"Yeah," I said, "but I want to look at everything that might be wrong and stay on top of the brand. So are you here all the time?"

"Nah," he said. "I'm always traveling around."

It's easy to say "Delegate!" but as it turns out, he runs around like crazy too. I think it's par for the course. If you're in business, no matter how much you delegate, if you want to be successful, you've got to stay on top of it. That's a very Spartan mindset.

Branson has moved beyond mere grit and determination. He's not forcing his way forward or making conscious effort to stay on track. He's doing what he loves, and as a result, it seems completely effortless and organic. He's not fighting; he's going with the flow. He is wired that way. He's doing what he loves to do. To me, Branson is the perfect embodiment of Spartan strength.

That's the state I want you to reach as well. At that point, you'll go home early from the party not as a sacrifice but because you *want* to be prepared in the morning to train. It's all for a much bigger purpose.

The boat ride was a frame-of-reference changer. It made the whole rest of the day that much more awesome. It put everything in perspective.

If you don't shift your frame of reference, if it becomes fixed and immutable, you become closed off to the magic and joy life has to offer, focusing instead on the trivial and inconsequential, inflating their significance to outlandish proportions because, after all, that's how you view the world. That weekend with Branson, I also encountered a rich woman who spent much of the time complaining about some mosquitos in the bathroom of the two-million-dollar villa she was staying in. You would think there would be no way you could complain in that situation, but if and when your frame of reference is your ten-million-dollar townhouse back in New York City, I guess you can.

You'll Know at the Finish Line

Branson lets his mind and spirit run wild and does a remarkable job of getting out of his own way. That's key, because the last obstacle you must surmount is the array of preconceived notions jammed into your psyche. All too often we spend our waking hours trying to find and stay comfortable in our own lives. We look for shortcuts, gadgets, and processes to make things easier, seeking what we consider personal fulfillment. We believe that there are things we can do and things that we can't, and we become conditioned to that distinction. It creates our everyday reality, and it makes us feel secure, because we think we know what to expect of the world and what to expect of ourselves. Sir Richard Branson hits the mute button on all of that negativity and focuses on what really matters, and the Spartan mentality helps you do the same.

This allows you to accomplish more than you ever thought possible. " 'You'll Know at the Finish Line' is a promise," says Spartan racer Tony Reyes. "A promise that if you work hard, dedicate yourself to your training, and give everything you have during the race, when you cross the finish line, you'll understand that who you were at the beginning of the race and who you are at the finish are completely different people. I know I am — don't you want to be?"

At the starting line, the racers psych themselves up one more time before hitting the course to test their mettle, but they're also celebrating. Simply getting to the starting line of the race is the start of the finish line. The feeling of exhilaration is hard to describe, but you see the sense of accomplishment etched on the faces of racers. As Tony mentions, we say you'll know at the finish line, yet you know certain things at the starting line, too. You pushed yourself off the couch, in many cases, and decided to change your life for the better. You were disciplined enough, in many cases, to prepare with months of training. You had the strength of character to show up and take your place at the starting line.

The gun sounds and all hell breaks loose. The rabbits, as they're called, bolt to the front. These racers — and every race has them — set an aggressive pace, but their ambitions outstrip their endurance, leaving them easy prey to more-patient, better-conditioned racers such as Kevin Giotti, who won five Spartan Races during the first half of 2012.

Kevin was doing the SoCal Super Spartan along with some buddies in 2011. A seasoned endurance athlete, he figured it would be a fun way to spend a morning and probably not terribly different from other obstacles races he had run. Only it was a bleak, gray day and unseasonably cold in southern California. The mountains at the racing venue were capped with snow, and rain was stopping and starting. What's more, the course was jam-packed with natural, as opposed to manmade, obstacles such as hills, washes, narrow single-tracks, steep ascents and descents, water, sand, mud, holes, weeds, trees, and rocks. Mother nature creates a mean obstacle course when she wants to.

"I had to run waist deep through twenty to thirty yards of water and, having emerged, jump over a fire line heavy with crackling flames and a big cloud of smoke," he recalls. "I charged up a wet, muddy, short-but-steep climb along a high ridgeline on a tight single-track that overlooked much of the venue."

Our goal, of course, was to pick up where mother nature had left off, making the course even harder. So the manmade obstacles would appear before Kevin one after the next: a javelin throw at a target; a long horizontal climbing wall; a bucket carry through cold water and back; a zigzagging balance beam; real, blood-drawing barbed-wire crawls very low to the ground; a twenty-five-yard tight tunnel crawl; a rope climb above water; heavy carry obstacles; and a Vaseline-rigged wall. No matter the obstacle, though, Kevin would have to keep pushing.

Then he came upon two truly unexpected obstacles that would throw him for a loop. A tire was hanging in the air, and he had to get through it. Do I dive through it or go feet first? he thought. As if that weren't enough, he had to stop and unlock a Rubik's Cube, too, while shaking with cold, muddy, and wet. The brain doesn't function well when the body is under siege, and Kevin's mind was as foggy as the shroud covering the mountains. Still, he figured it out.

For the rest of the day, as the later waves lined up to start in the corral, when asked how the race and course were, the best answer he could give was, "You have no idea what you've gotten yourselves into."

Kevin is now an elite Spartan racer, but it wasn't always that way. In 2001, he had just returned home from the world championship of an endurance event in Europe. He was out for a light training ride on his road bike when a moving van struck it from behind. The impact threw him sixty-five feet. His multiple serious injuries included thoracic spine fractures. It's hard to believe, but after a year of rehab, he was able to return to being an elite competitor.

This wasn't a race; it was a microcosm of life, taxing the brain and body alike in unexpected ways. Imagine the feeling of empowerment that comes from completing a race like this after having your spine crushed years earlier. That sort of accomplishment raises the bar on every other aspect of your life. You're not going to go back to a crummy job or a failing relationship or a crap diet and be content with that state of affairs. You now know that you can do so much better. No matter how impossible it seems, you can always reach your dreams.

"I haven't been the same person since I completed that first Spartan Race," says Kevin. "I knew when I crossed that finish line that it was only the beginning of a new-and-improved life." That's the Spartan ideal in action.

When I talk about having done three ultraendurance events in one week, you might think it sounds crazy. You might also wonder what it has to do with you. I'm not expecting you to want to mimic what I've done in the endurance field, even if you could. However, what I hope you do realize is that if I can do that — as crazy as it sounds — and it is crazy — then you can get up early enough in the morning to work out before taking your kids to school.

I mentioned before that once you think you're done running, you still have eight days left in you. The same goes for life. If you think you're maxing it out, you have no idea how much fuller and richer life could be. Spartan Race offers a glimpse into your own unlimited potential.

Quest for Fire in Your Belly

We believe that there are things we *can* do and things that we *can't*, and we come to accept that distinction. It creates our everyday reality, and it makes us feel secure, because we think we know what to expect of the world and of ourselves. Even if we're completely and utterly dissatisfied with life, it's a dissatisfaction that offers a certain degree of security. We know the rules, we know the boundaries, and we become comfortable being their prisoner.

Many people ask, "Why do a Spartan Race?" We heard it a lot when we were organizing our first Spartan Race in Vermont, and we still hear it today. There is no quick answer, or at least not one that is easily encapsulated in a sentence. I have to say it is the philosopher in me that continues to be drawn to obstacle racing as a sport. In the middle of a race, when all hell is breaking loose and your mind and body start to unravel, there is a revelatory wonder and sense of nowness that goes beyond what I can rationally express. And thus the irrational act of racing through mud and fire becomes rational. An insane behavior transforms itself into a very sane demonstration of human will. Spartan Race orchestrates for its racers the sense of wonder that is found in a kind of self-reliance that we seldom need in this society, where we have far more than we could ever use. Spartan Race forces you to awaken your senses. In the process, we begin to recapture what it feels like to be human.

This is what we mean when we say, "You'll Know at the Finish Line."

Vancouver, Washington, resident Heidie Bratlie needed her senses awakened in July 2010, when she weighed more than four hundred pounds. Determined to regain control of her body, she enrolled in a weight-management class. She was skeptical at first but put the dietary advice to work. The class taught her to avoid emotional eating, the trigger that had caused her to gain so much weight in the first place. After six months, she had lost more than one hundred pounds.

Then tragedy struck. Her husband, Jimmy, went in for what was supposed to be a simple surgery for carpal tunnel syndrome. They ended up finding another health problem, however, that killed Jimmy. "That was and still continues to be the hardest thing I have ever had to deal with emotionally," she says.

Rather than letting that tragedy derail her own progress, she kept exercising and eating well. Today she has lost 229 pounds. She'd heard about free workouts to prepare for a Spartan Race, and she decided to try one. Eventually she signed up for the Spartan Race scheduled for the summer of 2013 in Washougal, Washington. "I had no idea what I was signing up for," she laughs. "I had never heard of the Spartan Race but, like I said, I'm always up for a new workout."

"This year my goal was to finish, and I did that," she adds. "Now I have my sights set on next year. If everything goes as planned, I should be at my goal weight or very close, and I want to have even more fun, only faster than this year! The Spartan Race made me realize exactly how far I've come and also how far I have to go. I work hard every day. By next year, I will conquer!"

Heidi knows what the finish line means.

Many of the things I have written in this book may not harmonize with what you have heard your whole life. Nonetheless, I urge you to take my message and weigh it, consider it, and then begin to live it. People might say it's a ridiculous way of looking at life, or that it won't work, or that it's weird. Take heed when people say such things. It usually means that you're on the right path.

What's more, many of the people who will tell you to dismiss these ideas have reached a dead end on their own chosen path, whether they will admit it or not. The embrace of consumerism and convenience tends to lead to emptiness of the spirit and sickness of the mind and body. So the status quo isn't something to cling to. You were bombarded with these influences right after leaving the womb, and they have continued through childhood and adolescence and into adulthood.

My theory is that you need to rewire your brain to undo the constant onslaught of advertising and convenience and shortcuts that have been thrown at you for decades. The Spartan Race will definitely whip you into great shape. It can give you a tight butt or abs or pretty much whatever it is you want body-wise. But equally or more important, the Spartan lifestyle will help improve your mental strength and clarity of thought.

Everyone has to suffer to put things in perspective, and bitching burns between zero and zero calories a minute, so there's no use in complaining about your hardships. Think back to Sir Ernest Shackleton, the polar explorer whose ship became stuck in the ice in Antarctica. In Death Races, we have three days to make men and women feel like they would have felt being stranded in the ice with Shackleton on his adventure — except that lasted a year.

Out on the course, racers will say, "I'm so exhausted."

I'm like, "Yeah, Shackleton was tired, too."

"I'm so hungry."

"Yeah, so was he." I don't mention that he was so hungry that he ate his dogs.

These racers are so tired they can't see straight, they're speaking unintelligibly, and they're peeing themselves. They look at me and say, "Why do you keep telling me about some guy named Shackleton?"

I go: "Just think about what Shackleton went through. This is only three days. The guy was stranded with his men for nearly two years. He had no idea if he was going to live or die. You're going to live."

It's all in how you look at things. During another Death Race, someone said to me, "We are privileged." It didn't mean anything at the time, but now I realize: I am privileged. I have all my fingers, my toes, my arms. When you look upon the face of suffering, it recalibrates you. You realize how lucky you are that you don't have to deal with that every day.

Deciding to value our health and fitness does this, too; it helps us live life to the fullest. When you "Spartan Up!" it doesn't mean you are doing the most extreme endurance events. It's not about being a gym nut or being tougher than all your coworkers. It's about maximizing your life, realizing your greatest potential, and, in the end, living a memorable life. Spartan Up! is a change in attitude, which involves taking control of your life and your health.

Often you must hit rock bottom before you're ready to Spartan Up! While being athletic his whole life, Jeff Skowronski had also battled his weight, and more often than not he lost, until one day he looked down at the scale and saw 310 staring back at him. An approaching major life event would prompt him to set a short-term goal to lose some weight. For a while, he had some success. In one instance, his weight dipped all the way down to 244, a substantial loss of body fat. Yet after each such event, the weight returned. It became a vicious cycle.

When he became a father at age forty-one, Skowronski got serious about achieving weight loss that could be sustained for the long term. "If I wanted to walk my little girl down the aisle on her wedding day, I needed to make a change," he says. Living healthier wasn't enough of a goal for him, though; he needed something more concrete. So he decided to compete in a Spartan Race. In July 2012, he saw that a Spartan Sprint was scheduled in Pennsylvania in a few weeks. He finished that race and then another, a Super Beast in New Jersey, followed by a Beast in Texas, completing what we call a Trifecta. In Spartan speak, a Trifecta amounts to completing a Sprint, a Super, and a Beast in one racing season.

He recalls: "As I crossed the line in Texas, I had what I call a '*Biggest Loser* Moment,' and my eyes began to tear up. Here I was receiving my Trifecta. This was less than six months and forty-five pounds lighter, and when I thought that earning my Trifecta was impossible and something that only those amazing athletes on the cover of all the Spartan ads could do. Today I weigh 215 and have gone from a size 44 to a 36/34 waistline. By scheduling races regularly, I can't afford long breaks in my training or deviations from my diet."

Character and commitment such as that displayed by Jeff are not things people wear around their necks. They're invisible at first glance. How do you know that someone is trustworthy? How do you know what a person really believes? Sometimes only a rite of passage can show you. A rite of passage is an event marking a person's full inclusion in a social group. For instance, Masai males in Africa have to hunt and subdue a wild lion in order to be considered adults in the tribe. Marine Corps recruits suffer Death Race–level exertion and deprivation for over forty-eight hours before they receive their title and cap. Such rites of passage demonstrate that individuals have earned their place.

Day after day, I see people lacking any sense of place or belonging. They long to be part of something greater than themselves, something that's inspirational. We started out as a race company and we hold events. We are a business, but more than that, we are a community based on a certain way of life. On our website we provide a workout for the day, a training program, a food of the day, and other things that are part of a lifestyle, not just components of preparing for a race. People who visit our website want to know how we live.

People who make these choices want to go through something hard in life, and they want to do it while working in concert with others. But the rest of our society provides few opportunities for this. In America, we try to shield everyone from the pain of failure. When we're hurt, we look around for somebody to blame. When misfortune strikes, we look for somebody to sue. Kids get trophies for trying and losing because if they don't, the theory goes, they'll feel rotten about themselves. But out in the real world, they are ill equipped for the competition that they will face. They still think they will get a trophy just for good effort. Nothing could be further from the truth.

Failure creates a positive kind of pain. I experience this pain almost every single day. I set ambitious goals in my workouts, and most of the time I don't succeed. If I did 100 burpees without stopping yesterday, today I'll shoot for 110. Maybe I get 104 before my arms collapse. I failed, but you know what? That's okay. It's okay for me to fail. We all experience failure. This is what drives us to improve!

At the finish line, when a volunteer drapes a medal around your neck, a new chapter in your life has begun. Completing your first Spartan Race means that you have grit, toughness, and Spartan strength. You are someone who can be relied upon to complete the goals you set out to achieve. You've pushed yourself to a new level.

You're a changed person, part of a new community, and it's true what Tony Reyes said: Your life will never be the same.

Entering the Arena

One of my favorite quotes is from Theodore Roosevelt, who said: "The credit belongs to the man who is actually in the arena, whose face is marred by dust and sweat and blood, who strives valiantly; who errs and comes short again and again; because there is not effort without error and shortcomings; but who does actually strive to do the deed . . ."

Six-hundred-and-fifty thousand people of all backgrounds and with varying abilities have "entered the arena" and completed a Spartan Race. Nearly everyone who completes one seems to feel like they've started a new life in the process. I hear it all the time as people are leaving the venue or when they send me an e-mail afterward. They realize they are capable of finishing a demanding obstacle race, one that was designed to make them fail. As a result of this accomplishment, they believe they are capable of much more.

The Spartan Race has transformed along with its customers. We've come a long way from the early days, when races were held on a whim with little or no planning as challenge events for our friends and loved ones. We now orchestrate these heart-pounding events in the nation's largest sports stadiums, ski resorts, and elsewhere. As I mentioned earlier, obstacle racing is the world's fastest-growing sport after mixed martial arts.

Our "arenas" have gotten progressively bigger, and even the ancient Spartans might have been impressed if they had entered Fenway Park in Boston in November 2013 and seen racers scrambling up the stands en masse. This was a far cry from our first Spartan Race in Burlington, Vermont, with seven-hundred-some entrants.

The home of the Boston Red Sox had been transformed into a Spartan obstacle course for the second consecutive year. Twenty-two obstacles were dispersed across a 2.5-mile course for more than seven thousand competitors.

I had a few curve balls in store for the racers. Obstacles included hoisting a fifty-five-pound weight twenty-five feet into the air, pulling a rope hand-over-hand like a sailor hoisting a sail at sea. I couldn't tear up a Major League Baseball field to create mud pits, but I took full advantage of all those stairs, forcing racers to climb and descend them carrying forty-pound water jugs or sandbags rather than hot dogs and beer. I lined up rows of picnic tables and forced racers to scramble over them in succession. They also had to scale cargo nets, jump rope using heavy battle ropes, and push wheelbarrows up rickety ramps. As a final baseball-themed touch, I set up a "thirty burpees for fun" station on the outfield's warning track, the small strip of dirt between the grass and the fence.

Chikorita De Lego traveled from Mexico City to compete in that race. She's competed in both tae kwon do and soccer, but she's now an elite Spartan racer, our Mexican champion. She came to Boston to see how her elite status measured up among the American Spartans. Chikorita placed what was, for her, a disappointing fourth. She went back to Mexico, focused on improving her mental toughness, and, a month later, beat out Mexico's Olympian to take the top spot in the Guadalajara Spartan Race.

You won't find too many situations in life where people want you to push them harder than they've ever been pushed, where they're actually disappointed if you don't. If the course isn't hard enough, if it's not creatively masochistic, people will complain to me. I'm happy to push them so hard that they don't complain. Spartan Race wants you to achieve more. Hence we construct brutal and unforgettable courses. Our mission is to wow our racers, push their minds and bodies to the limit, and make them healthy through superior, extreme, and challenging obstacle races. That is why Spartan-brand obstacle race events are designed to break people down.

It hearkens back to a time when challenges weren't just endured; they were accepted and even welcomed. People passed the cookie test without realizing what it was; they just knew that if they made sacrifices now, the payoff would be greater later. Today, the opposite is true everywhere you look. You don't build a business for the long haul; you try to hit a quarterly number by hook or by crook. You don't build a championship team; you buy one through free agency. You don't pay your dues in the music business; you get on *American Idol* and succeed overnight.

These achievements ring hollow, because what matters is the journey, and there was no journey. Instant success imparts nothing of any real or lasting value. No adversity has been confronted and handled because everything came fast and easy. When adversity does arrive, and it always does, someone who has never encountered it before will have no clue what to do in response.

And so we keep erecting our obstacles, and we keep fighting through them to hone our skills and toughness. We're going to chip away at our goal of ripping seventy-eight million people off the couch and thrusting them into a healthy lifestyle. We aim to change people's lives by cultivating wellness and accomplishment at our events, through Spartan training, and in our online communities and by asking racers to lay their guts on the line and push their limits.

Everyone you've met in this book achieved something great because they didn't take the ultimate shortcut: instant gratification. The Spartan Races demonstrate what people can accomplish after making self-discipline a daily habit, rather than an isolated act or a New Year's resolution. Participants don't need to finish in first place or beat a particular time in order to triumph. Simply finishing is a great accomplishment. Having run a Spartan race, you'll go back to your job or family and solve problems more effectively because you'll see the path ahead differently. This new way of living is the difference between struggling and then dying unfulfilled or leading an epic life.

A fire burns within all of us, and we need an outlet to prove that we've got that fighting spirit. So I came up with this idea to create a race unlike any other race in the world, a race where nobody would know what to expect. In preparing for and then tackling one of our races, by proving that you can do it, you become a new person. Being a Spartan is about giving your best effort, proving your doubters wrong, and getting it done when other people are sitting at home watching TV. If you can handle a Spartan Race, you can handle anything else life sends your way, and that's true whether you're going blind, battling cancer, homeless, morbidly obese, or simply struggling to get through each day.

That's what you'll know at the finish line.

Living by the Spartan Code

Whether first-time racers or Olympic champions from other sports, all Spartan Race competitors are expected to meet an elite standard for sportsmanship. Race rules are posted on our website and at each event. All course rules are strictly enforced. Beyond race day rules, we promote the Spartan code to encourage and inspire Spartan Race participants and organizers alike to live up to the highest standards on race day and every day. According to our code:

- A Spartan pushes his/her mind and body to its limits.
- A Spartan masters his/her emotions.

SPARTAN UP!

- A Spartan learns continuously.
- A Spartan gives generously.
- A Spartan leads.
- A Spartan stands up for his/her beliefs, no matter the cost.
- A Spartan knows his/her flaws as well as his/her strengths.
- A Spartan proves himself/herself through actions, not words.
- A Spartan lives every day as if it were his/her last.

APPENDIX

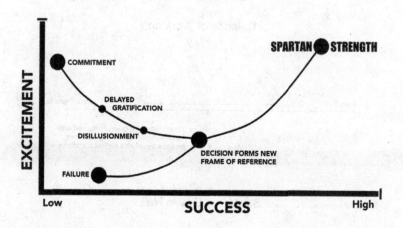

Appendix A: Road to Strength

A Spartan Theory of Happiness

A Day of Play Only

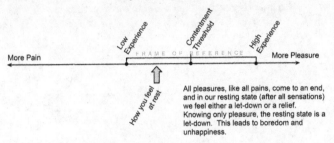

All pleasures, like all pains, come to an end, and in our resting state (after all sensations) we feel either a let-down or a relief. Knowing only pleasure, the resting state is a let-down. This leads to boredom and unhappiness.

Balance of Work and Play

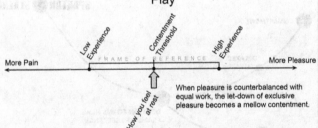

When pleasure is counterbalanced with equal work, the let-down of exclusive pleasure becomes a mellow contentment.

Start Your Day in Hell

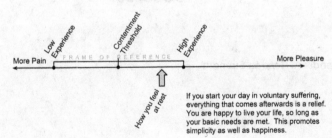

If you start your day in voluntary suffering, everything that comes afterwards is a relief. You are happy to live your life, so long as your basic needs are met. This promotes simplicity as well as happiness.

Appendix B: Frame of Reference

ACKNOWLEDGMENTS

Every Spartan Race is a collaboration among thousands of racers, a thousand or more spectators, hundreds of volunteers, and a few dozen other helping hands. While this book convened a far smaller group of contributors, it was also a highly collaborative endeavor, and a number of these individuals deserve recognition.

You met many of my family members in the book. Among them, a big thanks to: My parents, Ralph De Sena and Jean De Palma. They helped make me who I am today. Without them and their heartfelt encouragement, I would be on an entirely different path in life, one that wouldn't have been nearly as fun as this one.

My aunts and uncles, too numerous to single out here, who reinforced all the lessons I absorbed from my parents. They too deserve a big aroo!

My wife, Courtney De Sena, who deserves the biggest thanks of all for letting me be a Spartan every day. I knew she was the one for me the moment we met, and my instincts were right. She is an amazing and integral part of Spartan Race and my life.

Our children, Jack, Charlie, Catherine, and Alexandra. Running Spartan Race "the business" and running other people's endurance events as a competitor already takes me away from them more than I wish were the case, so I appreciate the additional sacrifices they endured as I was writing this book.

My sister, cousins, and close friends. All of them have enriched my life in some profound way.

My second family is my Spartan crew, many of whom were instrumental in helping bring the Spartan story to life, whether it was offering insights for the book or keeping the ship sailing as I was writing it. I'd like to thank the following:

Jason Jaksetic, who runs the Spartan Race "Workout of the Day" and "Food of the Day" factory in Vermont.

Mike Levine, who provided me with helpful notes throughout the process.

Kari Glasier, who offered me insights, particularly with respect to the concept of transformance.

Carrie Adams, who was instrumental in fleshing out "You'll know at the finish line" as a concept and rallying cry.

The Jains, who help me every day with the business and just navigating planet Earth. Their help on this book was par for the obstacle course.

Al Cappucci and Marty Fox, who make sure our Spartan ship is always sailing in the right direction, even when the seas are choppy and the winds change. Sir Ernest Shackleton may be my hero, but better not to lose your way in the first place.

David Michael DeLuca, an indefatigable researcher who tracked down quotes, studies, and anything else I needed to flesh out my ideas and concepts. I couldn't have completed this project without his Spartan determination and diligence.

Raptor Consumer Partners, the private-equity firm that got behind Spartan Race when funding was the big obstacle looming ahead.

The folks over at Reebok, who stepped it up and took the plunge by backing this new sport based only on our vision and a handshake.

And everyone past, present, and future at Spartan Race headquarters.

I also want to thank those non-Spartans who helped with the creation of the book:

Jeff O'Connell, who found a way to turn my Queens slang into English and helped craft a book that captures the Spartan ethos. He spent countless nights working on it, on the heels of his day job as editor-in-chief at Bodybuilding.com, and for that I am grateful.

Marc Gerald at the Agency Group, for believing in the story and bringing it to an outstanding publisher who supported the project, Houghton Mifflin Harcourt.

Susan Canavan at Houghton Mifflin Harcourt, for acquiring the proposal and guiding the manuscript to completion with such skill and insight. Her assistance during the process helped give shape and form to an array of people, places, events, and ideas that might have overwhelmed a lesser editor. We would never have reached the finish line of this endurance event without her encouragement and patience.

Martha Kennedy, for designing the jacket in Spartan style; and Brian Moore, for making the book's interior shine.

Anne McPeak, for copyediting the manuscript, even though she made us do thirty burpees for every misspelled word.

Jeff Gomez of Starlight Runner Entertainment, for reading the manuscript with such a discerning eye and offering such perceptive insights.

Thanks to Jaloyn, "the ultimate Spartan" who pushed through no matter what the task.

A final thank-you to Spartan racers everywhere:

To those whose stories and experiences are somehow relayed or referenced in this book: thank you for letting us share your story with the world. All of you embody the essence of the Spartan Race, and I'm proud to have included you.

To the hundred of thousands of Spartans who have done our races but who aren't mentioned in this book: thank you for trusting us and believing in our mission. By doing a Spartan Race, you are not only changing your own life but you are making it possible for others to change their lives. Without your leadership by example and support, we would not exist. Thank you for paying it forward.

Congratulations on your purchase of

SPARTAN UP!

Use code "**SPARTANUP15**" at checkout
and save **15%** on any U.S. Spartan Race.

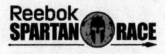

www.spartan.com

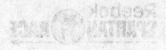